12-14-72

Dear Bob.

Your help was invaluable during the production of the [...] ope you will be plea [...] complimentary cop [...]

Merry Christmas,

Jack.

THE TROPHIC FUNCTION
OF
LYMPHOID ELEMENTS

THE TROPHIC FUNCTION
OF
LYMPHOID ELEMENTS

By

JACK W. SHIELDS, M.D., M.S., F.A.C.P.

Department of Medicine
Santa Barbara Medical Clinic and the Cottage Hospital
Santa Barbara, California

With a Foreword by

J. M. Yoffey, D.Sc., M.D., F.R.C.S. (England)

Department of Anatomy
The Hebrew University
Hadassah Medical School
Jerusalem, Israel

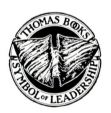

CHARLES C THOMAS • PUBLISHER
Springfield • Illinois • U.S.A.

Published and Distributed Throughout the World by
CHARLES C THOMAS • PUBLISHER
BANNERSTONE HOUSE
301-327 East Lawrence Avenue, Springfield, Illinois, U.S.A.

© *1972, by* CHARLES C THOMAS • PUBLISHER
ISBN 0–398–02412–X
Library of Congress Catalog Card Number: 74–175087

With **THOMAS BOOKS** *careful attention is given to all details of manufacturing and design. It is the Publisher's desire to present books that are satisfactory as to their physical qualities and artistic possibilities and appropriate for their particular use.* **THOMAS BOOKS** *will be true to those laws of quality that assure a good name and good will.*

Printed in the United States of America
EE-11

To

PAT, MARK, and JONATHON

FOREWORD

IT GIVES ME great pleasure to write a foreword to *The Trophic Function of Lymphoid Elements*. Dr. Shields and I have shared for many years a common interest in the lymphocyte and the lymphomyeloid complex. To the best of my recollection this interest dates from well before the great lymphocyte explosion which burst upon the biological world just over a decade ago. At a time when, strange as it now may sound, lymphocytes were "mature" cells deserving but scant attention, Dr. Shields and I would meet at scientific gatherings, and in between the formal sessions would settle down to off-the-record discussions of our differences of opinion, which were, and still are, profound.

The problems presented by that "Cellula Plena Mysterii," the lymphocyte, have been aptly compared to the pieces of a gigantic jigsaw puzzle. While it is true that in recent years some of the pieces in this puzzle have been fitted into place, the puzzle as a whole still has extensive gaps remaining to be filled. In an effort to fill these gaps, Dr. Shields has over the years been engaged in bold and far-reaching speculations. In the formulation of his views he has read widely, and has not hesitated to challenge many time-honoured concepts.

I feel sure that most readers will join issue with Dr. Shields in some of the points which he makes in this book. I feel equally certain that the book will stimulate them to think again about some matters which they had previously regarded as settled. From what I know of Dr. Shields, the success of the book in evoking second thoughts will be the reward which he most desires.

J. M. YOFFEY
The Hebrew University
Jerusalem

vii

INTRODUCTION

THIRTY-SIX YEARS ago, Dr. Arnold Rich [1] stated: "Regarding the lymphocyte, I am sure that all who are engaged in the study and teaching of pathology will agree that the complete ignorance of the function of this cell is one of the most humiliating and disgraceful gaps in all medical knowledge." Fourteen years ago, Dr. O. A. Trowell [2] concluded his comprehensive but succinct review on lymphocytes quoting the same statement.

At almost the same time Dr. Rich's provocative statement was published, it was found that lymphoid cells, such as plasmacytes and medium-sized lymphocytes, produce antibodies. (Earlier it was believed that reticuloendothelial cells, particularly macrophages, are the source.) Since Dr. Trowell's seconding of Dr. Rich's statement, it has been established that following appropriate sensitization, small lymphocytes can (a) transform into antibody-producing cells in tissue culture, (b) destroy tissue transplants from other individuals, (c) retain immunologic memory for specific antigens for many years, and (d) transfer specific immunologic reactivity from one individual to another. Although it remains to be settled how lymphocytes become sensitized and how they carry forth some of these functions, many have concluded that the primary function of lymphocytes is an immunologic one. Consequently, to modify immunologic reactions toward transplanted tissues, to maintain and enhance defense against pathogenic microorganisms, and to learn more about natural immunity in neoplastic conditions, unprecedented funds and effort are being expended each year, both publicly and privately, in basic and applied research on lymphocytes.

Some time before Metchnikoff, von Behring, von Pirquet, Landsteiner, and many others laid the foundations for modern concepts of immunology, and even longer before immunology became recognized as an exacting, applied science, anatomically oriented individuals such as Hunter, Hewson, Dionysius, and Ranvier set forth observations indicating that the fundamental function of lymphoid cells is to feed other cells in the body. Relatively modern physicians such as Carrel, White, Kelsall, Crabb, and Loutit have presented additional observations to support this point of view. Because of the circumstantial nature of the evidence presented, the feeding or trophic concept of lymphoid tissue and lymphocyte function remains to be considered seriously by contemporary physicians, biologists, and others potentially interested in how growing cells within the body are nourished.

My primary purpose here is to present, review, and correlate data indicating that the basic function of the lymphoid elements, including lymphoid organs, lymph, lymphocytes, and other mononuclear cells, is indeed trophic. Secondarily, the data will be organized to indicate that the currently recognized immunologic functions of these elements are also important aspects of this feeding function. In this light, immunologic functions will be envisioned as sophisticated mechanisms by which foreign, genetically incompatible, or spurious matter are destroyed, thus reducing them into relatively simple substrates which can be reutilized conveniently for growth in an individual's cells. Thus, through an immunologic capacity to destroy foreign proteins and foreign living matter, the latter will be removed from a position where they are toxic to, or feeding upon, the body fluids and cells of the host to a status wherein they can be utilized as food within host cells.

My interest in this subject started some 15 years ago during the course of a morphologic study [3] on the blood and hemopoietic organs of a series of individuals afflicted with relatively obscure hematologic diseases. The study involved differential counting of more than 120,000 nucleated blood cells, as well as the gross and microscopic evaluation of the organs from which they were obtained. During this exercise, the mass, tremendous numbers, and variety of lymphoid elements to which the various hemopoietic organs give rise were most impressive. The discrepancy between the complement of such elements in the lymphoid organs, as compared with microscopically visible counterparts in the circulating blood, was also impressive. Subsequent study and research on the lymphoid organs and lymphocytes of humans and small animals (see Table I) has led me to believe that Dr. Rich's statement still remains painfully true. This may be owing to the

TABLE I
MATERIAL EXAMINED*

Human:	*Marrow*	*Nodes*	*Spleen*	*Thymus*	*Intestine*
Lymphoma	10	15	8		
Hodgkin's disease	2	10	5		
Myeloma	19	0	3		
Reticulum cell sarcoma	2	2	5		
Acute leukemia	15	0	0		
Chronic leukemia	13	1	10		
Polycythemia vera	3	0	2		
Myeloid metaplasia	15	0	14		
Megaloblastic anemia	7	0	0		
Hemolytic anemia	45	0	15		
Hypoplastic anemia	25	0	1		
Iron deficiency	30	0	0		
Granuloma	3	11	3		
Lupus erythematosus	4	0	3		
Felty's syndrome	3	0	4		
Portal hypertension	0	0	5		
Thrombocytopenic purpura	15	0	10		
Traumatic rupture	0	0	3		
Miscellaneous	71	61	0		
Normal	77	0	0		
Removed incidental to:					
1. Esophagogastric surgery			8		3
2. Mastectomy		111			
3. Bowel resection		69	2		69
4. Plastic surgery		8			
Capsule biopsy					8
	359	297	101	0	80
Guinea pig (adult): Healthy	0	8	8	8	8
Starved	0	6	6	6	6
Rat:					
One day	0	2	2	2	2
Three weeks	0	3	3	3	3
Three months	0	3	3	3	3
Twelve months	0	2	2	2	2

* The human series includes specimens obtained 1965 to 1967 at the Santa Barbara Medical Clinic and specimens obtained 1950 to 1956 at the Mayo Clinic (see Refs. 3, 53, 68, 80, 111).

consideration that relatively few people are aware of the contributions of early and contemporary anatomists as they apply to the mass of clinical and experimental data which has accumulated in very recent years. Therefore, normal and developmental anatomy will be stressed during the ensuing thesis on the trophic function of lymphoid elements.

ACKNOWLEDGMENTS

I SHOULD LIKE to express my gratitude to Dr. M. M. Hargraves and Dr. Gertrude Pease, under whose guidance this study commenced in 1955 in Rochester, Minnesota. Also my thanks are given to a host of helpful colleagues, lay personnel, and private patients at the Mayo Clinic, Rochester, Minnesota; the Field Clinic and the University of Illinois School of Medicine, Chicago, Illinois; and the Santa Barbara Medical Clinic and the Cottage Hospital, Santa Barbara, California. I am indebted to the late Dr. Dameshek and to the Editorial Staff of *Blood,* the Journal of Hematology, for constructive criticism during preparation of portions of the manuscript; to Dr. George Halling of the Santa Barbara Medical Clinic for collaboration on the section dealing with the endocrine function of the thymus; to Drs. Wilton Doane and James McKittrick of the Santa Barbara Medical Clinic for continuing help in obtaining fresh surgical material for study; to Dr. Delbert Dickson of the Cottage Hospital Pathology Department for help with the preparation, study, and special techniques applied to this material; to Drs. Robert Touchon and Michael van Buskirk, medical residents at the Cottage Hospital, for help with the differential counting of cells in tissue sections; and to Drs. Marianna and Francis Masin, Cytology Consultants to the Santa Barbara Medical Clinic, for stimulating discussion and help with significant references. Also, I appreciate the help of a group of diligent secretaries, including Anne Forslund, Hazel Adams, Betty Gillingham, Olive Bailey, and Nancy Morris; and the help of cooperative librarians, including Mrs. Elizabeth Perry, Margaret Tully, and Miss Elizabeth McChristie.

Finally, substantial assistance from the Santa Barbara Medical Clinic Research Fund should be acknowledged.

CONTENTS

SECTION 1
THE TROPHIC FUNCTION OF VARIOUS
LYMPHOID ELEMENTS

SECTION 2

THE TROPHIC FUNCTION OF THE THYMUS
AND SMALL LYMPHOCYTES

SECTION 3

ON THE INTRAVASCULAR SECRETION OF
BLOOD AND LYMPH

SECTION 4
CONCEPTS NEW AND OLD

THE TROPHIC FUNCTION

OF

LYMPHOID ELEMENTS

Section 1

THE TROPHIC FUNCTION OF VARIOUS LYMPHOID ELEMENTS

The lymphoid elements, including the lymphoid organs, lymph, lymphocytes, and closely related mononuclear cells, characteristically reside, for the most part, between the peripheral tissues and the circulating blood.[4,5] Being closely related to both, one must consider their orientation toward each.

Chapter 1

THE RELATION OF LYMPHOID ELEMENTS
TO THE CIRCULATING BLOOD

THE BLOOD IS a liquid medium which flows through vessels to carry water, oxygen, and various kinds of nourishment to the tissues. In humans it consists of plasma and formed elements in a ratio of approximately 55 to 45 percent.[6] The term "plasma" is generally used to describe the slightly turbid, colorless fluid which remains after the formed elements have been separated out; whereas the term "formed elements" is ordinarily used to describe the erythrocytes, leucocytes, and thrombocytes normally suspended in the circulating plasma. The plasma and formed elements together, in the form of whole blood, normally constitute 7 to 8 percent of total body weight.[6] Both the plasma and the formed elements arise embryologically from mesenchyme scattered throughout the body of the embryo. As the vessels develop from mesenchyme, however, the continued production of blood becomes localized primarily in definitive blood-forming organs concerned with the production of specific types of blood elements (see Sect. 3). The blood-forming organs are known as hemopoietic or hematopoietic organs (although the term "heme" refers only to the red pigment which imparts to blood its distinctive color and its relatively great capacity to carry oxygen). Blood, nevertheless, consists of many substances besides heme.

The hemopoietic organs are subdivided into myeloid and lymphoid systems, each of which normally comprises 1 to 2 percent of total body weight.[6-9] It is generally recognized that the myeloid (marrow-like) system produces the bulk of the formed elements in the blood, including the erythrocytes, granulocytes, and thrombocytes, which in terms of volume constitute more than 99.5 percent of the formed elements.[6]* It remains to be

---

* Lymphocytes normally account for the small remainder of formed elements and normally constitute one-fourth to one-third of the leucocytes in the blood.[6]

recognized that the lymphoid system produces the bulk of the plasma and the lymphocytes which are secreted in the form of lymph † via lymphatics into the blood vascular system. Moreover, it remains to be recognized that the lymphoid system augments the trophic, as well as immunologic, function of the blood by producing plasma and lymphocytes.

---

† It is significant etymologically that the term "plasma" is derived from the Latin *plasma*, meaning something formed or molded—hence, a formed substance. The derivation of the term "lymph" is more complex. This term is derived from the Greek νύμφη, meaning nymph. By the obvious association with water, this probably merged into the Latin terms *limpa, limpidus*—hence, limpid, referring to clear, or pure, water. The Latin terms *lympha* and *lymphaticus* were originally used to connote states of madness or frenzy. In the subsequent text, the word lymph will be used to describe the colorless or white fluid in lymphatics—a fluid normally consisting of plasma wherein variable numbers of lymphocytes are suspended.

Chapter 2

THE MASS AND GROWTH RATE OF LYMPHOID ELEMENTS

IN HIGHER EVOLUTIONARY forms of animal life which breathe air and possess bony skeletons which enable them to walk on land, the myeloid component of the hemopoietic system uniformly resides quite remote from the external environment within the various bones and drains its products directly into the systemic venous system. The lymphoid component of the hemopoietic system, on the other hand, is located diffusely in areas of the body both close to, and remote from, the external environment and drains its products into the blood circulation indirectly via lymphatics, or via the portal venous system.[7,8] Together, the lymphoid organs, lymph vessels, and lymph have been called the "lymphatic apparatus" by Drinker and Yoffey.[7,8] The apparatus includes the lymphoid organs, such as the spleen, lymph nodes, thymus, periarteriolar lymphoid tissue of the bone marrow, the diffuse and nodular lymphoid tissue underlying the mucosal surfaces of the intestine, the lymphatic vessels serving the former, and the lymph contained in the lymphatics. Excluding the vessels and the lymph which they contain, but including the lymphoid cells which are scattered throughout the connective tissues and epithelia, the total lymphoid tissue mass is estimated, as already mentioned, to constitute 1 to 2 percent of total body weight [7-9]—a tissue mass roughly equal to that of the active (red) bone marrow, the liver, or the brain. Owing to their relatively small size, e.g. one-third to one-tenth that of liver cells or cortical neurones, the lymphocytes no doubt constitute the most common nucleated cells in the body of the healthy individual.

It is characteristic of the lymphoid organs and the lymphocytes which normally make up 80 to 90 percent of their component cells that they have a normal propensity to grow at an exceedingly rapid rate, as compared with the cellular components of the liver, brain, remaining body tissues, and even the bone marrow. For instance, first, on the basis of mitotic indices (the rate of mitosis per given numbers of cells), it is calculated that the rate of cell renewal in lymphoid tissues and particularly in lymphocytes is sufficiently rapid to double the number of lymphocytes in the body every 48 hours in healthy animals.[9-12] Second, in the lymphoid tissues, particularly in lymphocytes, the rate of DNA precursor utilization, an index of the cellular growth rate, far exceeds that in remaining tissues of the body[13,14] (see Sect. 2). Third, sensitivity to x-irradiation, another guide to cellular growth rate, is approximately ten times as great in lymphoid tissues as in remaining tissues of the body.[15] Under ambient conditions of atmospheric oxygen tension and barometric pressure, approximately 5000 rads of x-irradiation are required to kill the bulk of cells in most parenchymal tissues. Individual tissue sensitivity may be increased by hyperbaric oxygenation or peroxide infusion and may be decreased by anoxia or reducing agents, such as sulfhydril compounds.[15] Under ambient, or standard, atmospheric conditions, 50 rads of local or total body radiation is sufficient to induce chromatolysis (fragmentation of nuclear chromatin) in the small cytoplasm-poor lymphocytes found in the thymic cortex and in the follicles of remaining lymphoid organs.[16] The most radiosensitive target appears to be the phosphate bonds in the nucleotides of their nuclear deoxyribonucleic acid (DNA).[16-18] Under the same conditions, doses of 500 rads of total body radiation will induce almost complete lymphocytolysis (fragmentation of lymphocytes) and disappearance of lymphocytes throughout the follicles and medullary reticulum of the spleen and nodes, the reticulum of the thymus, and in the reticular connective tissue of the gastrointestinal submucosa, leaving only the less radiosensitive histiocytic and undifferentiated stromal elements in all these areas.[15] From the latter, new lymphocytes are generated when the dose is sublethal.[15] Close to and above 500 rads (the median lethal dose in most mammals), in conjunction with extensive lymphocytolysis and consequent atrophy of the lymphoid tissues, there ensues a syndrome characterized by

anorexia, nausea, diarrhea, rapid wasting, and profound immunologic paralysis. In doses significantly greater than 500 rads of
total body radiation, death usually follows unless bone marrow
or lymphoid tissue transplantation is successfully accomplished.[15]
Even then, immunologic paralysis and wasting take place, particularly in newborn animals (see Sect. 2).

Such observations on the mass and growth rate of the lymphoid
tissues, together with the wasting and immunologic paralysis which
supervene when this mass is destroyed, have led some, such as
Loutit,[19] to suggest that the lymphoid component of the hemopoietic system plays an important role in nutrition, as well as in
immunology.

Chapter 3

PHYSIOLOGIC VARIATION IN THE LYMPHOID TISSUE MASS

THE LYMPHOID TISSUE mass estimate of 1 to 2 percent of body weight is based on observations in animals feeding normally, free from infection or trauma, and not under stress immediately prior to sacrifice.[7-9] Infection usually induces enlargement of the lymphoid organs in the region of the site of infection. Starvation and stress induce rapid shrinkage of the entire lymphoid tissue mass, with the loss of weight being particularly well documented and striking in the thymus, spleen, and intestinal lymphoid tissue.[7,8,20-24] Starvation for three days induces at least 58 percent loss of wet weight in the intestinal lymphoid tissue [25] and 35 percent loss of dry weight in the spleen.[26] Within 4 to 5 hours after realimentation, the intestinal lymphoid tissue is restituted and 24 hours after, this has occurred with the splenic mass.[24-27] With each meal containing protein, or protein and fat, the intestinal lymphoid tissue and spleen rise sharply in mass and then shrink between meals.[25-27]

The loss of mass induced by starvation or stress is largely due to the disappearance of small lymphocytes—a loss which is not compensated for by their appearance in increased numbers in the blood or lymph, or as intact cells in other tissues.[7,8,22-24] During stress it is clear that the small lymphocytes undergo lysis *in situ* and usually begin to do so within minutes after the stressful episode.[22-24] Although some of the nuclear material subsequently undergoes phagocytosis in the lymphoid organs,[7,8,24] it is not clear what happens to all the products of lymphocytolysis or what useful purposes they serve after release. During starvation, the rate of disappearance of small lymphocytes and loss of organ weight is slower than during conventional forms of stress, such as hemorrhage, exposure to cold, operative procedures, fright, etc. It is not clear whether during starvation the small lymphocytes disappear from the lymphoid organs by lysis, by emigration coupled with lack of replacement, or both.

In addition to the variation in mass which occurs during stress, starvation, and infection, the lymphoid tissue mass varies with age. The mass is poorly developed in all areas except the thymus gland at the time of birth.[7-8,28-29] It reaches its largest total mass in proportion to total body weight near the time of puberty (interestingly enough when the basal metabolic rate reaches its highest point during life).[7,8,28,29] The lymphoid tissue mass shrinks gradually in relation to total body weight with senescence.[7,8,28,29] For such reasons, the true size of the lymphoid tissue mass is difficult to assess at necropsy, as most individuals die as a result of aging, infection, starvation, or as a result of more than one of these entities. Only in purposeful sacrifice or in sudden accidental death is the normal size of the lymphoid tissue mass fully appreciable.[30]

Undoubtedly, it was observations on the variation of this mass with feeding and its large size during the period of rapid body growth which led early anatomists such as Hewson,[31] Hunter,[31] and Dustin [32,33] to propose that the lymphoid organs and lymphocytes play an important role in nutrition and in general body growth.

Chapter 4

THE CELLULAR COMPOSITION OF THE HEMOPOIETIC ORGANS

THE BONE MARROW and lymphoid organs consist internally of an embryonal type of stroma wherein various kinds of blood cells develop.[4,5,34-44] This blends into the bony or fibrous stromata which supply their external form and their structural support, respectively. This intrinsic stroma has the physical consistency of gelatin with varying degrees of firmness, depending, perhaps, on the state of hydration.[45] Owing to the fact that it is traversed by many fine argentophilic (silver staining) fibrils, this gelatinous stroma is called the reticulum (from the Latin diminutive of *rete,* meaning a net—hence, a fine network).[36,40,41] It consists of syncytially arranged mesenchymal mononuclear cells whose relatively abundant cytoplasm contain the fine fibrils, commonly known as reticulin [36,40,41] (and see Sect. 3). The relatively amorphous cytoplasm, reinforced by such fibrils, constitutes the matrix or ground substance in which the various types of blood cells are supported and receive nourishment as they grow.[4,5,34-44] Relatively differentiated components of the reticulum associated with or producing relatively large numbers of fibrils and coarser fibrils are commonly recognized as fibroblasts.[34-46] Relatively undifferentiated components of the reticulum producing relatively few, if any, fibrils are designated as reticular cells (or reticulum cells).[4,5,34-46] Such elements are believed to constitute the adult counterpart of embryonal mesenchyme.[4,5,34-46] From the latter are differentiated various types of myeloid cells in the marrow and lymphoid cells in the lymphoid organs, either directly or by the intermediary formation of large precursor cells called blasts, e.g. erythroblasts, myeloblasts, megakaryoblasts, monoblasts, plasmablasts, and lymphoblasts.[4-6,36,40,41,47]

Although there remains no unanimity of opinion concerning the identity, individual developmental potential, and mode of

differentiation of all kinds of blasts,[6,47] particularly the lymphoblasts,* it is characteristic of each and every hemopoietic organ to
give rise to a variety of blood cells. During embryogenesis in
lower orders of vertebrates and in mammals afflicted with certain
diseases, the lymphoid organs produce erythroyctes, granulocytes,
and thromboyctes, as well as monocytes and lymphocytes.[48,50]
The mesenchymal portion of the liver, for a period of time
during embryogenesis, produces most of the blood cells of all
kinds and during adult life in mammals remains capable of resuming formation of myeloid, as well as lymphoid, elements.[48,51]
Into adult life, as myelopoiesis evolutes in the marrow cavities,
the mammalian marrow continues to produce relatively large
numbers of monocytes, plasmacytes, and lymphocytes, along with
the characteristic myeloid elements.[52,53] The relative numbers
of different types of blood cells normally produced in various
human hemopoietic organs (as well as their relative oxygen requirements for growth in relation to the vasculature) are sche-
matically outlined in Figure 1a, b.

From the various hemopoietic organs, blood cells or their cytoplasmic products are decimated into the circulatory system in
characteristic forms, i.e. as whole cells (granulocytes, monocytes,
lymphocytes), as cells whose nuclei have disintegrated or have
been extruded (erythrocytes), as cytoplasmic fragments (thrombocytes), or as fragments of cells too small to be identified microscopically, as in the free extracellular proteins shed from plasmacytes and other mononuclear cells (see below). It is undoubtedly owing to the variety of forms in which they are
secreted into the blood that the term "formed elements" instead
of "cells" is used to describe the microscopically visible elements
in the circulating blood. Whole blood nevertheless is a composite
of the former, together with free extracellular proteins and the
water which allows the composite to flow through vessels to
carry oxygen and various kinds of nourishment to the tissues.

---

* For this reason, and because the developmental potential of the small lymphocyte will be seriously questioned, the term "lymphoblast" will not be used to
describe a stage in lymphocyte development. Instead, the term "large lymphocyte"
will be used. In the plural, the term "lymphoblasts" will be reserved for use as it
translates literally, i.e. as precursors of lymph.

Large numbers of fixed and motile mononuclear phagocytes are found in the hemopoietic organs of all species, closely associated with the reticulum wherein the formed elements are derived and supported prior to their release into the blood or lymph stream.[34-54] These phagocytes, known as histiocytes and macrophages, are found not only in the extravascular reticulum but also in the lining of vascular channels known as sinusoids [41,43,44,54] (see Sect. 3). Normally these cells do not appear as intact cells in the circulating blood.[6] Instead, they live out their life span and perform their useful functions in close relation to the reticular stroma. Although Ranvier [55] considered these cells to be elements (clasmatocytes, see below) which shed their cytoplasm for the nutritive benefit of other cells, most consider them (after Metchnikoff) [56] to be concerned primarily with the ingestion and the disposition of endogenous and exogenous particulate matter, therefore primarily concerned with immunity. Such interpretations are not necessarily mutually exclusive, as we shall see later.

The reticulum of the hemopoietic organs also contains tissue mast cells and fat cells.[57,58] The latter are found primarily in the marrow,[58] whereas the former are found throughout the hemopoietic organs.[58] The role of the fat cells in storing lipids which can be mobilized for nutritional purposes is well known. It seems significant that during prolonged starvation, fat cells disappear throughout the loose connective tissues of most body organs, but increase in number within the marrow cavities to replace hemopoietic elements.[57] The relative number of tissue mast cells in the hemopoietic organs and loose connective tissues appears to fall during starvation and rise with adequate protein nutrition.[58]

Finally, the hemopoietic organs contain arteries, veins, lymphatics, and sinusoids which are characteristic of hemopoietic organs in general and characteristic within each definitive kind of hemopoietic organ (see Fig. 1b and Sect. 3). These vessels not only carry into the hemopoietic organs the substrate from which blood is to be manufactured and carry away the formed elements which have been produced, but also do so in patterns, which are specifically oriented centrally and peripherally in the different hemopoietic organs.

Chapter 5

THE ORIENTATION OF HEMOPOIETIC ORGANS TOWARD VESSELS AND OTHER ORGANS

I N ADULT MAMMALS, the myeloid component of the hemopoietic system grows within various bones, receives the substrate necessary for cell growth entirely from small nutrient
arteries of the bones, empties its cellular products entirely into
small systemic veins, is devoid of lymphatics,[7,8] and is thus isolated
from the body surfaces in contact with the external environment. Simply, the bone marrow is oriented exclusively toward
the blood vascular circulation and, through the latter, toward the
tissues in general. On the other hand, the lymphoid component of
the hemopoietic system is made up of diverse organs, each of
which is characteristically oriented, directly or via lymphatics
either toward body surface or toward specific vital organs.[7,8] (See
Figs. 1–3 which summarize this graphically.)

A. LYMPHOID COMPONENTS OF THE HEMOPOIETIC SYSTEM

a. Intestinal Lymphoid Tissue

The intestinal lymphoid tissue is characteristically oriented
toward the mucosal lining of the gastrointestinal tract, which
is concerned with the production of digestive enzymes and the
absorption of food. In the small intestine where the bulk of
absorption takes place, one normally finds the bulk of the
gastrointestinal lymphoid tissue.[7,8] This lymphoid tissue can be
subdivided into three components (see Fig. 3a).

First, the diffuse submucosal lymphoid tissue immediately
underlies and directly supports the mucosal cells,[34] especially in
the small intestinal villi (where the bulk of absorption takes
place). This lympoid tissue receives the substrate necessary for
growth more or less directly from the absorptive cells, as well as

17

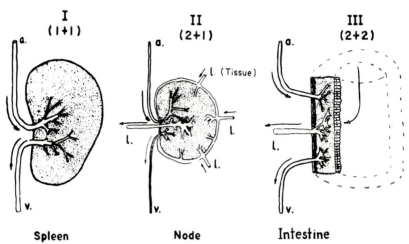

I
(1+1)

II
(2+1)

III
(2+2)

Spleen   Node   Intestine

Figure 2. Some of the subdivisions of the lymphoid tissue mass grouped according to afferent substrate supply. It will be noted that the spleen is supplied primarily by an afferent artery (a.) and drains via an efferent vein (v.). The nodes, in addition, are supplied via afferent lymphatics (l.) and drain via efferent lymphatics (l.). The lymphoid tissue of the intestinal submucosa (stippled), in addition to arteries (a.), is supplied with substrate newly absorbed via the mucosal cells and drains via lymphatics (l.) as well as veins (v.). From Shields, J.W.[98]

from tiny arterioles. It empties its formed cellular products into tiny, centrally oriented lymphatics called lacteals.*

Second, the nodular submucosal lymphoid tissue is dispersed

---

* Whereas the formed cells and free extracellular products of lymphoid tissues generally emigrate via lymphatics into the systemic venous circulation, newly absorbed free amino acids and low-molecular-weight fats largely migrate to the liver via the portal venous system.[7,8,34,59,60]

Figure 3a. A detailed diagram of the intestinal lymphoid tissue showing primarily the location of the lymphoid tissue and the lymphatics. At levels a-b are found the lacteals and diffuse lymphoid tissue of the intestinal submucosa (stippled in the central third of the lower third of the lower portion of the diagram). At levels b-d (above are found the nodular lymphoid tissue of the submucosa (Peyer's patches) and the plexus of lymphatics which supply and drain the nodules. Below level g, on the mesenteric side of the intestine, is shown a mesenteric lymph node which interrupts the central flow of lymph emanating from the diffuse and nodular lymphoid tissue of the intestinal submucosa. From Kampmeier, O.F. (see Reference 7, Section 3).

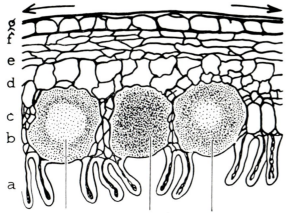

g
f
e
d
c
b
a

lymph nodules of Peyer's patch

intestinal lumen

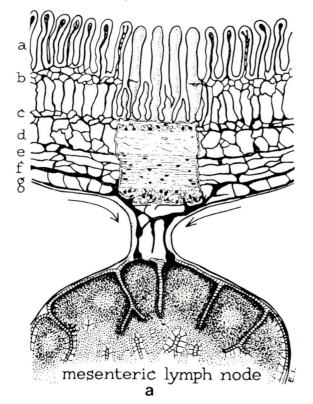

a
b
c
d
e
f
g

mesenteric lymph node

a

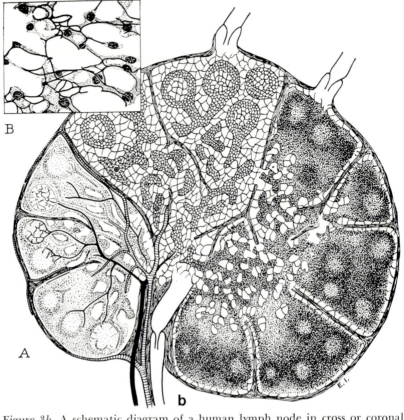

Figure 3*b*. A schematic diagram of a human lymph node in cross or coronal section, cut through the hilus. In A (approximately x 6), the right half of the figure indicates the disposal of the lymphoid tissue into cortical nodules and medullary cords; the middle part, that of the connective tissue framework after removal of the lymphocytes; the left part, that of the blood vessels (cross-lined and black) entering and leaving via the hilus. Afferent lymphatics are seen entering the node above and the efferent leaving at the hilus, their valves indicating the direction of flow. Inset, B (after Heidenhain), pictures a minute part of the framework, greatly magnified, to show the network of reticular (reticulum) cells and their supporting fibrils (black). Relatively dense stippling in the (outer) cortex of the node represents a relatively dense homogeneous population of small and medium-sized lymphocytes embedded in relatively dense reticular stroma. (Compare the right and middle third of diagram A). The pale, lightly stippled areas in the cortex represent germinal centers. The dark, densely stippled areas immediately surrounding the germinal centers represent the mantle zones, consisting mostly of small cytoplasm-poor lymphocytes. Where the densely stippled and densely reticulated architecture of the cortex fades gradually into the looser, more sparsely stippled medulla, are found the perifillicular, or paracortical portions of the node. From Kampmeier, O. F. (see Reference 7, Section 3).

irregularly through the gut but largely in the distal small intestine where the bulk of protein absorption takes place. This lymphoid tissue receives the substrate necessary for cellular growth at successively greater distances from the mucosal cells either via the lacteals or via small systemic arterioles. It empties its cellular products primarily into centrally oriented lymphatics in the mesenteries.[7,8] *see,* also, footnote p. 18.

Third, the mesenteric nodes are dispersed in mesenteries, especially in the mesentery of the small intestine. These nodes receive the substrate necessary for cell growth either from the centrally oriented lacteals or centrally oriented lymphatics previously mentioned and from the mesenteric arterioles. They empty their cellular products primarily via central lymphatics into the thoracic duct.

The central lymph emanating from these three segments of the intestinal lymphoid tissue (all primarily oriented toward the absorptive mucosal surface of the gut) constitutes the bulk of the lymph transmitted via the thoracic duct into the central arteriovenous circulation, the quantity varying directly with the amount of protein, or protein and fat, absorbed during the previous meal.[7,8]

b. Lymph Nodes

The lymph nodes are characteristically oriented toward almost each and every definitive organ in the body but are located at varying distances from these organs and are clustered as regional nodes in relatively specific locations alongside the arterial supply of the organs in question. The regional nodes are so situated that all lymph draining from the periphery (peripheral lymph) passes through them before draining centrally via central lymphatics into the paired cervical and thoracic lymph ducts which, in turn, drain into the arteriovenous system at the base of the neck.[7,8] The regional nodes are thus specifically oriented toward diverse organs. They receive the substrate necessary for cellular growth both from these organs via peripheral lymphatics, and from their intrinsic arterial supply. They empty their cellular products primarily via central lymphatics into the central arteriovenous circulation by means of the paired cervical and thoracic lymph ducts.

c. Spleen

The spleen is characteristically oriented on its afferent aspect toward the arterial circulation via a single relatively large artery known as the splenic artery. On its efferent aspect, it is oriented toward the liver via the splenic vein which drains into the portal venous system. Lymphatics are generally lacking in the spleen, except in the adventitia of its larger vessels and in its capsule.[7,8,41] In the spleen, therefore, the substrate necessary for cellular growth is received entirely from the large splenic artery. Its cellular products are emptied largely into the liver via the portal system and must pass through another capillary bed there before gaining access to the general circulation, either via hepatic venous blood or via lymph effluent from the liver. In its orientation, the spleen differs from remaining lymphatic organs in that it is oriented primarily toward the liver on its effluent aspect, rather than toward the lymphatic or systemic blood circulation. On its afferent aspect, being oriented only toward the arterial circulation, it is oriented purely toward the cellular output of the bone marrow and toward the circulating output of remaining lymphoid organs.

d. Thymus

The thymus is characteristically oriented toward clusters of epithelial cells embryologically stranded from the primitive gill system and toward small afferent arteries in the upper thorax. Lacking afferent lymphatics, the thymus receives the substrate necessary for cellular growth entirely from the latter, but the rate of its cellular growth may be greatly affected by secretions from the former (as will be emphasized in Sect. 2).

e. Periarteriolar Lymphoid Tissue of Marrow

The periarteriolar lymphoid tissue of the bone marrow is characteristically oriented toward the tiny nutrient arterioles of the marrow cavities. As lymphatics are normally lacking in the marrow,[7,8] this component of the lymphatic apparatus is obliged to receive the substrate necessary for cellular growth from the tiny nutrient arterioles and must empty its cellular products either into the marrow at large or into the venous effluent of the marrow.

As will be brought out in Chapter 11, these various forms of specific orientation undoubtedly have a great deal to do with the patterns of cellular growth and function in various components of the hemopoietic system.

Chapter 6

THE ARTERIAL SUPPLY OF HEMOPOIETIC ORGANS

ALL BODY ORGANS receive water, oxygen, and various forms of substrate essential to the growth and function of component cells by means of their afferent arteries. Some organs are more generously supplied with arteries and their ramifications than others, but the hemopoietic organs exemplify the extremes. Whereas the bone marrow is sparsely supplied by nutrient arteries of bones; the lymphoid organs are richly supplied with arterial blood via single or multiple arteries of caliber relatively large in relation to the volume of tissue into which they ramify.[53] Upon entering the lymphoid organs, the arteries ramify extensively into arterioles whose numbers in cross section are relatively great as compared with the bone marrow and most non-hemopoietic organs.[53] As true veins are not demonstrable in the lymphoid nodules where the arterioles are largely concentrated and wherein many lymphocytes are generated,[61] it is not clear how blood actually flows through lymphoid organs to gain access to veins, or else filters into efferent lymphatics. Currently advocated is that the arterial blood flows entirely through "closed" vessels lined entirely by endothelium; but some maintain that, in part, it flows directly into and through the reticulum via "open" channels lined by other kinds of cells (see Chap. 16 and Sect. 3). Regardless of the pathways involved, quantitative differences in the arterial blood supply have important physiologic consequences in the hemopoietic organs. For instance, in the bone marrow, where the arterial supply appears relatively poor, the tissue oxygen tension resembles that of systemic venous blood (e.g. partial pressure of oxygen on the order of 40 mm Hg).[62] Relatively low oxygen tension, in turn, is conducive to the growth of myeloid elements, especially erythrocytes, which normally develop beside venous sinusoids remotely located from

24

the sparsely dispersed marrow arterioles.[52,53,57] Lymphoid elements in the marrow characteristically grow in a periarteriolar location [52,53] (see Fig. 1a and b).

Second, in the lymphoid organs where the arterial supply is relatively rich, the tissue oxygen tension approaches that of arterial blood [53] (e.g. 100 mm Hg). Relatively high oxygen tension, in turn, is conductive to the growth of lymphocytes [63] which normally develop in periarteriolar locations throughout the hemopoietic system [53] (see Figs. 1–3, which summarize this graphically).

Finally, owing to the fairly rich arterial blood supply, in addition to oxygen, the lymphoid organs are supplied with relatively large quantities of substrate which can be utilized for DNA synthesis and cellular growth at rates which are rapid compared with those in the marrow and in many other organs of the body (see Chap. 16).

Chapter 7

THE LYMPHOCYTES AND OTHER
MONONUCLEAR CELLS

IN THE ADULT mammal, it is characteristic of the bone marrow to produce a variety of cells whose nuclei either become segmented or disappear before the cells (e.g. leucocytes) or their products lacking nuclei (e.g. erythrocytes and thrombocytes) are released to become the common, microscopically visible, formed elements in the circulating blood. The term "polymorphonuclear" (many forms of nucleus) literally describes such formed elements derived from the marrow; but the term is generally used to characterize those leucocytes (white cells) which normally develop specific granular organelles (tiny organs) in their cytoplasm during maturation. The polymorphonuclear leucocytes include the neutrophilic, eosinophilic, and basophilic leucocytes which, on the basis of the affinity of their cytoplasmic granules for certain aniline dyes, are called neutrophilic, eosinophilic, and basophilic granulocytes, respectively.

On the other hand, the lymphoid organs produce cells whose nuclei remain ovoid or round, regardless of the state of maturation, the presence of specific cytoplasmic organelles, and where these cells are found, whether in the bone marrow or lymphoid organs, in the circulating blood or lymph, or in other tissues. Since they are relatively lacking in the colorful, granular organelles, some of these cells have been called nongranular leucocytes. More commonly, they are called mononuclear (one nucleus) cells. Included among the mononuclear cells are the reticular cells (fine net cells), histiocytes (tissue cells), macrophages (big eaters), monocytes (single or singular cells), plasmacytes (form or mold cells), and lymphocytes. The last were probably so named because they constitute the most common type of cells in lymph and in lymphoid organs. (For a schematic estimate of the relative numbers of these cells, their relative size,

26

and their relative relationship to the vasculature in various hemopoietic organs, see Fig. 1b).

Unfortunately, there remains no unamimity of opinion concerning the precise definition of each kind of mononuclear cell, the precise criteria which should be used to differentiate one from another, or precisely how they are interrelated, particularly in terms of genesis and function.[47] In very gross but not necessarily universally acceptable terms, the reticular cells may be identified by their integral position in the reticular stroma (see Sect. 3); their ovoid, reticular (skein-like), pale-staining nuclei of maximal diameter of 12 to 14 μ in Wright's stained smears, or 8 to 11 μ in 10% formalin-fixed, hematoxylin- and eosin-stained sections; and the relative lack of specific organelles or fibrils in their abundant pale-staining cytoplasm. The histiocytes and macrophages may be identified under the same conditions by their reticular nuclei of similar size but more variable shape, and slightly denser chromatin. Their relatively abundant cytoplasm, under the light microscope, stains pale and may contain visible particles which have been ingested (usually the partially digested remnants of other types of cells). Under the electron microscope, it contains relatively large numbers of cytoplasmic lysosomes. The monocytes may be identified by their somewhat smaller, seldom round, but similar nuclei; and their somewhat less abundant, pale-staining, but dusty cytoplasm which seldom contains visible foreign particulate matter under the light microscope; and which contains relatively abundant lysosomes under the electron microscope.

The plasmacytes may be identified by their relatively round nuclei whose chromatin is relatively coarse and dense and whose nuclear diameter ranges from 6 to 25μ. Their fairly abundant cytoplasm is deeply basophilic with Wright's stain or pyroninophilic with methyl green pyronin; or demonstrates relatively large numbers of ribosomes and well-developed endoplasmic reticulum under the electron microscope. Normally such cells lie closely associated with relatively large numbers of definitive plasmacytes with eccentric nuclei and paranuclear halos, as described by Von Marschalkó (see below).

The lymphocytes in their large, immature stages may be identified by criteria similar to those already mentioned with respect to the larger plasmacytes but are generally found in close association with, or surrounded by, relatively large numbers of very small mononuclear cells. The round nuclei of the latter, ranging from 5 to 10μ in Wright-stained smears or 4 to 8μ in fixed tissue sections, are extremely dense with coarsely blocked chromatin. Their scant, variably basophilic cytoplasm contains relatively few organelles of any specific kind. The latter type of small cells, by differential counting, normally constitute 80 percent of the cells in the spleen, 90 percent of the cells in the lymph nodes, perhaps 95 percent of the cells in the thymus, and 70 to 90 percent of the mononuclear cells in the circulating blood and lymph of mammals.[3,6-8,35,64-68]

Beyond the relative numbers of small lymphocytes, the numbers of other mononuclear cells in the hemopoietic organs remain open to argument, partly owing to problems surrounding precise classification and partly owing to the fact that differential counts in aliquots sampled but subjected to examination by different techniques (e.g. Wright-stained smears, hematoxylin- and eosin-stained sections, pyronin-stained sections, and electron-microscopic sections) may yield differing results. In Wright-stained smears of aspirates or imprints (the standard hematologic technique whereby the cells were originally described and continue to be classified), differential counts of nucleated cells reveal that in normal adult bone marrow, granulocytes, erythroblasts, and megakaryocytes account for 87.4 percent of the cells; whereas the remaining 12.6 percent is made up of reticular cells (0.2%), monocytes (2.0%), plasmacytes (0.4%), and lymphocytes (10%).[6] More than three times this percentage of any of the latter is probably abnormal.[6] Of the 3 to 17 percent (average 10%) of the lymphocytes normally found in human marrow (as compared with the spleen), a relatively high percentage will be found to be medium-sized lymphocytes (nuclear diameter 11–14μ—cells which are often called "transitional lymphocytes." Large lymphocytes (nuclear diameter 15–25μ) are seldom recognized as such in normal marrow, where germinal centers are lacking.

In normal adult human splenic aspirate, segmented granulocytes (owing to hemodilution) make up 25 percent of nucleated cells. The remaining 75 percent consist of reticular cells (0.1%), macrophages and histiocytes (0.1%), monocytes (2.0%), plasmacytes of the von Marschalkó type (0.2%, see p. 76), large lymphocytes (0.1%), medium-sized lymphocytes (5.0%), and small lymphocytes (65–70%).[68] Normal adult human lymph nodes contain a smaller percentage of granulocytes, reticular cells, histiocytes, macrophages, monocytes, and plasmacytes; a small percentage of medium-sized lymphocytes; and a larger percentage of small lymphocytes than the spleen. It is characteristic of the normal thymus to exceed the nodes in all these parameters. In the normal intestine, the diffuse lymphoid tissue in the submucosa resembles the bone marrow with respect to a relatively high percentage of plasmacytes and medium-sized lymphocytes, whereas the nodular lymphoid tissue (Peyer's patches) and the mesenteric nodes more closely resemble the lymph nodes in general.

As pointed out by Downey,[36] it is characteristic for the nuclei of the reticular (or reticulum) cells to *enlarge* as they "round-up" to become stem cells or "blasts" for different kinds of formed elements. In the marrow, as differentiation and mitotic division of the "blasts" proceed, it is characteristic for the nucleocytoplasmic ratio of the bulk of elements thus differentiated to *fall,* so that with increasing maturation of granulocytes, erythrocytes, and thrombocytes, the portion occupied by the nucleus becomes progressively smaller (as in granulocytes) or disappears (as in erythrocytes and thrombocytes). On the other hand, in the lymphoid organs, it is characteristic for the nucleocytoplasmic ratio of the cells differentiated from the "blasts" to *rise,* so that with increasing maturation of lymphocytes, the portion of the cell occupied by the nucleus becomes progressively larger.

Thus, in attempting to assess the function of myeloid elements, one must look primarily toward the cytoplasm. But in attempting to fathom the function of lymphoid cells, one must look chiefly toward the nucleoplasm (see Sect. 2), and toward the cytoplasm which has disappeared (see below and Sect. 3).

Chapter 8

THE KINETICS OF LYMPHOID ELEMENTS

THE TERM "KINETICS" literally means "movements." As the lymph, blood, and hemopoietic organs are more purely and obviously in a state of flux than remaining tissues in the body, this term is commonly used to describe the sites and rates of production, the patterns of migration, and the sites and rates of disappearance of different kinds of blood elements. Hence, the terms "erythrokinetics," "granulocytokinetics," "thrombocytokinetics," and "lymphokinetics" are popular. The last term, however, is not ordinarily used to describe the movements of lymph as a whole but only the movements of lymphocytes. The assessment of kinetics of the various blood elements is made by sampling the blood, lymph, hemopoietic organs, and other organs at prescribed intervals of time with a view toward the cell as a whole or with a view toward some component in the cell which can be marked or labeled specifically and thus traced.

Irrespective of where it is sampled, the circulating blood has a relatively uniform concentration of water, salts, plasma proteins, plasma, and formed elements, the quantities of each remaining relatively constant with respect to one another.[6] The arterial blood differs from venous blood principally in its higher oxygen, higher glucose, and lower carbon dioxide concentration. On the other hand, lymph varies greatly in consistency, depending upon where it is sampled.[7,8] It resembles arterial blood in that it has a relatively high oxygen and low carbon dioxide concentration[69] but differs from the blood in general in that it contains no erythrocytes, platelets, or granulocytes, and generally contains a concentration of lymphocytes higher than that of blood.[7,8] Its free extracellular protein concentration is always lower than that of blood, and its albumin:globulin ratio always higher.[7,8] In general, its concentration of lymphocytes and its concentration of proteins rise, while its concentration of water and its albumin:globulin ratio fall as one samples lymph progressively closer to its point of entry into the arteriovenous circulation via the paired thoracic and cervical lymph ducts.[7,8] The peripheral lymph which flows from all peripheral tissues to regional nodes contains relatively few cells and relatively little free extracellular protein, especially globulin. The central lymph which flows from the nodes into the thoracic and cervical lymph ducts contains a relatively high but variable concentration of lymphocytes, a higher but variable total protein concentration, and a higher concentration of globulins than peripheral lymph.[8,7,70] The portal venous effluent of the spleen contains a higher but variable concentration of lymphocytes and a higher concentration of oxygen than systemic venous blood.[71] Only the lymph effluent from the liver contains relatively few lymphocytes and a protein concentration and albumin:globulin ratio approaching that of circulating blood.[7,8]

Such findings can be explained on the basis that the lymphoid tissues actively secrete lymphocytes and free extracellular proteins, particularly globulins, into lymph as it proceeds from the periphery toward the central arteriovenous circulation (see below) ; or on the basis that the capillary beds vary in permeability to proteins and cells, the peripheral capillary bed being least permeable, the capillary bed in the nodes being more permeable, and the capillary bed in the liver being most permeable.[7,8] It remains to be recognized that each explanation may be partially correct.

While it is generally recognized that the lymphoid organs produce very large numbers of lymphocytes, the actual rate of production remains open to question because calculations based on mitotic indices in lymphoid organs and lymph catheterization data are at variance with calculations based on data obtained by isotope labeling and chromosome marking (see Chap. 16, E) . On the basis of the catheterization data, it is calculated that sufficient lymphocytes leave the lymphoid organs and migrate via the thoracic duct into the blood circulation to replace all the lymphocytes in the latter 2 to 12 times daily (depending on the species) .[7,8] Additional, but unknown, numbers of lymphocytes enter the blood circulation via the right thoracic duct, the paired cervical lymphatic ducts, the portal venous effluent of the spleen, and probably via the venous effluent of the marrow. On the basis of mitotic indices, it is calculated that 2.8 times as many lymphocytes are produced daily by the total lymphoid tissue mass as enter the bloodsteam via the thoracic duct.[12] Calculations thus yield a daily replacement factor (DRF) of circulating blood lymphocytes on the order of 2.8 times 2 to 12, and sufficient (in humans) to replace all the circulating blood lymphocytes every one to two hours.[12] On the other hand, on the basis of isotope-labeling data and chromosome-labeling data, it is calculated that 30 to 60 percent of the circulating blood lymphocytes are cells of prolonged biologic life which are not newly formed lymphocytes, but lymphocytes of long biologic life which continuously recirculate from blood to lymph via the lymph nodes (see Chap. 16, E). Such discrepancy between the results obtained by the different methods of calculation remain to be explained.

Similarly, it is generally recognized that the lymphoid organs secrete free extracellular proteins into lymph, particularly globulins known as immunoglobulins capable of agglutinating a host of specific antigens and that these globulins are of relatively short biologic half life in the blood (e.g. 2–21 days).[72,73] However, it remains to be settled:

1. Precisely how lymphoid cells secrete these free extracellular proteins.
2. How much they actually secrete normally.
3. Precisely what kind of lymphoid cells secrete which free extracellular proteins.
4. How these free extracellular proteins are utilized and disposed normally, as well as during immunologic and disease processes.

Owing to the fact that the rates of production are not clear and the mode of disposition of the cells and their free extracellular products remain to be settled, the lymphokinetic data remains incomplete.

A singular discrepancy in blood cell kinetics appears to lie in the volume of elements secreted from the lymphoid component of the hemopoietic system in comparison with that secreted from the myeloid component. The bone marrow, whose total active mass (as red bone marrow) is estimated to be 1200 to 1500 gm in the healthy 70 kg human, normally maintains some 2100 cc (4+ pints) of formed elements in the circulating blood.[6] As it remains to be recognized that the lymphoid organs secrete large quantities of plasma or plasma proteins, the lymphoid tissue mass (estimated to be 700 to 1400 gm in the 70 kg adult) is acknowledged to maintain merely 8 to 12 gm (2–3 teaspoons) of lymphocytes in the circulating blood.[42] Thus the lymphoid tissue mass exceeds the mass of its known secretory product in the circulating blood by a factor of 50 to 200, whereas the active marrow mass is actually exceeded by the mass of its secretory products which include the erythrocytes (replaced in the blood every 100 days), granulocytes (replaced every 4–8 hours), and thrombocytes (replaced every 4 days).[6] While it is recognized that the lymphoid organs also secrete free extracellular proteins in the form of immunoglobulins, the latter normally constitute less than 10 percent of the plasma proteins (whole total mass is on the order of 350 gm).[72-77] The discrepancy between lymphogenous and myelogenous production becomes even more striking but complex when one considers on the basis of the isotope data (see Chap. 16) that the lymphoid component of the marrow appears to produce lymphocytes more rapidly than the remaining lymphoid organs (with the possible exception of the thymus) and that in the paraproteinemias wherein the production of specific immunoglobulin classes is excessive, most of the excess appears to emanate from abnormal cells in the marrow.[6]

Finally, in terms of literal kinetics, distinctive forms of pure movement within the body are displayed by lymph and lymphocytes. Characteristically, the latter, particularly the small cytoplasm-poor lymphocytes, are endowed with a capacity for active and independent motility which far exceeds that of remaining cells in the body, including the granulocytes, monocytes, and macrophages.[2,78] By virtue of this capacity, the small lymphocytes (having migrated more or less passively within the blood and lymph streams) are empowered to move through the endothelial

TABLE II
CLASMATOSIS

Year	Author	Cell Type	Significance Accorded	Material Studied
1844	Donné		Secretion of globulines	Lymph
1890	Ranvier	Macrophages ("Clasmatocytes")	Secretion of nutrients	Omentum
1900	Dominici	Spleen Cells	Shedding of platelets	Human spleens
1907	Renaut	"Cellules Rhagiocrines"	Secretion of cytoplasmic products	All tissues
1912-1913	Downey and Weidenreich	All mononuclear cell types in lymphoid organs	1. Secretory process 2. Process whereby small lymphocytes are formed	Human and small animal lymphoid organs
1922	de Assua	Plasmacytes	Secretory process	Small animals
1939	Sabin	Macrophages ("Clasmatocytes")	Secretion of antibodies and other proteins	Peritoneal exudates
1943-1946	White and Dougherty	Lymphocytes	1. Secretion of immune and normal globulins 2. Nutritive	Small lab animals
1949	Leitner	Plasmacytes	Secretion of paraproteins	Human marrow
1953	Englebert	Thymocytes		Tissue culture
1961 1964 1966	Shields	All mononuclear cell types in lymphoid organs and marrow	Secretion of plasma	Humans and small animals
1969	Rondonelli et al.	Large mononuclear cells	Process whereby small lymphocytes are formed	Tissue culture of newt tails

cells (plasmacytes) in lymphoid organs rather than from macrophages.

As a result of clinical studies on human bone marrow, Leitner [95] suggested that myeloma cells (immature plasmacytes) secrete paraproteins (certain classes of immune globulins produced in abnormally great quantity) by shedding cytoplasm (see Figs. 53 and 54). With the application of phase-contrast microscopy and time-lapse microscopic cinematography to tissue culture systems, several subsequently described cytoplasmic shedding from lymphocytes as it occurs *in vitro*. Describing the process as it is accelerated by glucocorticoids and alluding to Downey and Weidenreich's early observations, White and Dougherty [20-23] concluded (1942–1953) that lymphocytes secrete normal, as well as immune, globulins by shedding cytoplasm and by undergoing total lysis. White [21] suggested further that the lymphoid organs perform important nutritive functions in so doing. Studying thymocytes (thymic lymphocytes) growing in tissue culture, Englebert [96] in 1953 concluded that many of these cells shed cytoplasm during differentiation. In 1961, 1964, and 1966, evidence was correlated to indicate that the various kinds of mononuclear cells subserve an important nutritive function by shedding cytoplasm to create plasma, which in turn carries nutrients as well as formed elements to the tissues.[97-99] Although unconcerned with the fate of the shed cytoplasm, Rondanelli *et al.*[100] showed recently that larger mononuclear cells obtained from newts transform in tissue culture into small lymphoid cells by cytoplasmic shedding.

As the magnitude as well as physiologic significance of such cytoplasmic shedding remains to be generally appreciated, Figures 4 to 27 are included to illustrate various aspects of the phenomenon as observed in hemopoietic tissues fixed* promptly after their removal from living subjects.

---

* Tissue fixation involves the precipitation of protoplasmic and extracellular proteins by fixatives such as alcohols, aldehydes, organic acids, or heavy metals, so that the tissue cells will lose their gelatinous consistency and become firm enough to maintain shape on glass slides or withstand embedding in solid media for slicing into histologic sections. The fixation process usually results in 10 to 40 percent dehydration and shrinkage of the tissue cells, the amount of shrinkage being roughly proportional to their water content. Prompt fixation is desirable in order to avoid artefacts owing to migration of motile cells, autolysis of stationary cells, and various degenerative changes which take place with time after death or removal of cells, tissues, and organs from their natural habitat.[34]

Figures 4, 5, and 7 to 26 (specimens obtained from the marrow and lymphoid organs of healthy humans or small animals) show that various kinds of mononuclear cells shed cytoplasm in the form of tiny droplets or globules. The droplets are found in progressive states of demarcation and separation from the peripheral cytoplasm of the cells (Figs. 4–12 and 15–27). In addition, myriads of separate droplets are found adjacent to and between the cells (Figs. 4–12 and 15–27). On shedding from the cells, many of the droplets appear to undergo progressive changes, including hyalinization,* decreasing basophilia, disintegration, dissolution, and final dispersion into the pale blue background which consists of precipitated plasma and other extracellular proteins (see Figs. 4–12). As contrasted with the myriads of droplets found in the interstices of lymphoid organs, relatively few are found in the efferent lymphatics (see Figs. 9 and 10) or thoracic duct (Fig. 26), and practically none are found in the circulating blood—either separating or separate from the cells. Such a decremental distribution, together with the progressive morphologic

---

* This tinctorial change presumably reflects depolymerization of cytoplasmic proteins during change of state from gel to sol. Owing to this hyaline appearance, Downey and Weidenreich referred to the droplets as hyaline bodies.

→

Figure 4. Medium-sized lymphocytes shedding cytoplasmic droplets (arrows). Normal human lymph node aspirate; Wright's stain × 1200.

Figure 5. Macrophage (A), large lymphocyte (B), and medium-sized lymphocytes (C) shedding cytoplasmic droplets. Separated droplets between the cells (dots). Normal guinea pig spleen imprint; Wright's stain × 1200.

Figure 6a. Malignant hematopoietic cells shedding droplets (arrows). Human bone marrow aspirate; reticulum cell sarcoma, stem cell type; Wright's stain × 1200. Note fragmentation and dispersion of droplets into the less basophilic background.

Figure 6b. Same situation as in Fig. 6a but from a different patient. Note the large numbers of basophilic droplets between cells and their disintegration, dispersion, and dissolution into the background.

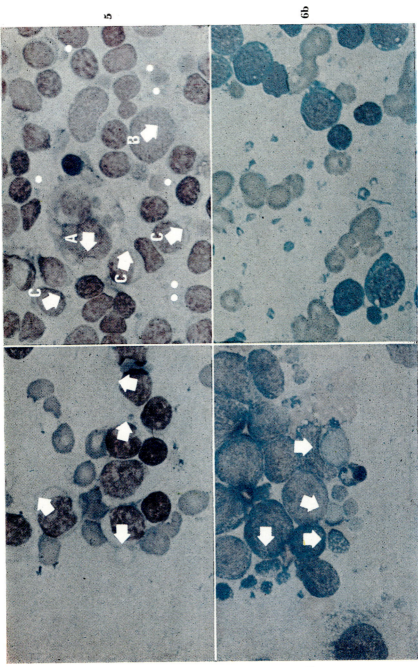

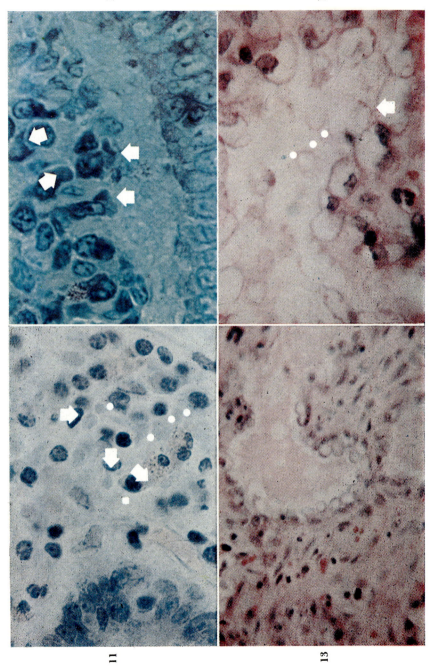

12

14

11

13

whether it be in smears, imprints, or tissue sections. In the bone marrow, where the ratio of medium-sized to small lymphocytes is relatively high normally, cytoplasmic shedding is found routinely in medium-sized lymphocytes, but these cells are relatively few in number as compared with erythroblasts and granulocytes. The myeloblasts also appear to shed cytoplasm (as noted by Downey),[86] but once specific granules commence to appear in cytoplasm, the propensity to shed disappears. Thus, shedding is unusual in granulocytes differentiated beyond the progranulocyte (promyelocyte) stage.

In specimens obtained from healthy subjects, histiocytes and macrophages appear to shed cytoplasm in prolific fashion while engaged simultaneously in the digestion of visible particulate matter (see Figs. 5, 21, and 22). Normally, however, such phagocytes are numerically uncommon in comparison with medium-

←

Figure 11. Core of human small intestinal villus with mucosal cells to the left and a lacteal (space) centrally. Cytoplasmic droplets shedding from medium-sized lymphocytes and plasmacytes (arrows). Separated droplet in the lacteal (square dot), and other separated droplets in the interstices (round dots). Tissue obtained by jejunal tube biopsy; 2% glutaraldehyde fixation; hematoxylin and eosin stain × 1200.

Figure 12. Core of normal rat intestinal villus with mucosal cells below. Cytoplasmic droplets shedding from plasmacytes (arrows). Two percent glutaraldehyde fixation; aqueous May-Grünewald-Giemsa stain × 1200.

Figure 13. Lactating human breast. Cytoplasmic droplets shedding from apical portion of mammary epithelial cells and dissolving to yield milk within the duct. Ten percent formalin fixation; hematoxylin and eosin stain × 400.

Figure 14. Lactating human breast. Cytoplasmic droplets shedding from the mammary epithelial cells. Ten percent formalin fixation; hematoxylin and eosin stain × 1200.

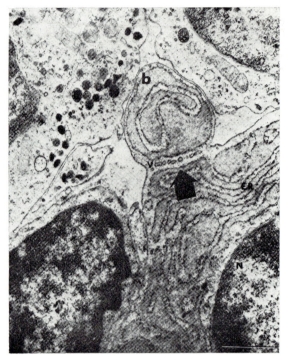

Figure 15. Cytoplasmic droplet (b) starting to shed from the peripheral cytoplasm of a marrow plasma-cyte × 21,600. From Goodman and Hall.[135]

sized lymphocytes in all hemopoietic organs (but are relatively common in the liver; see Fig. 1b).

Droplet shedding from plasmacytes does not appear to be so prolific as compared with that from medium-sized lymphocytes of similar size, but owing to the intense basophilia of their cytoplasm, the droplets emanating from plasmacytes are relatively easy to identify (see Fig. 12). Plasmacytes, as defined by von Marschalkó (see below), are relatively uncommon in normal hemopoietic organs (except the diffuse intestinal lymphoid tissue). Thus, large and medium-sized lymphocytes in healthy subjects remain the most common source of cytoplasmic droplets.

Also, in specimens obtained from healthy subjects, study of the nuclei of cells shedding cytoplasm will reveal that most show no evidence of chromatolysis or any other degenerative change which

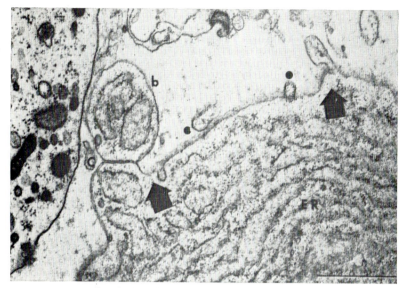

Figure 16. Cytoplasmic droplet (b) starting to shed from a marrow plasma-cyte. Smaller droplets separating, or separated at the superior margin of the cell (dots) × 41,500. From Goodman and Hall.[135]

distinguishes them from adjacent cells which do not appear to be shedding (see all figures). This finding led Downey and Weidenreich [36,86-88,101] to conclude that cytoplasmic shedding is not indicative of a degenerative process but a *secretory* process. It is relatively common, however, to find some mononuclear cells resembling small and medium-sized lymphocytes whose nuclei show various states of chromatolysis and whose cytoplasm is obviously disintegrating into tiny amorphous fragments. Throughout the hemopoietic organs, such disintegrating cells are relatively common, both as isolated elements and as elements which have undergone partial digestion within histiocytes and macrophages. No absolute figures on their relative frequency are available because most pass them over as "damaged" or "fragile" cells and fail to include them in differential counting. One may estimate that their number as isolated cells (not within phagocytes) is on the order of 1 to 5 percent of the mononuclear cells in most of the hemopoietic organs. Their significance will be considered subsequently in Section 2.

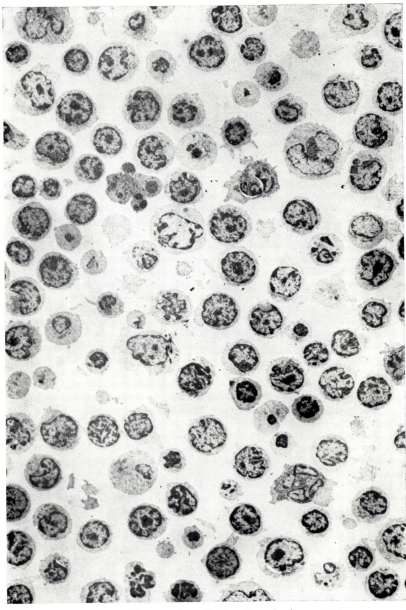

Figure 26. Human throacic duct lymph; low-power electron photomicrograph × 2,900. Many cytoplasmic droplets between the cells. Although many of their nuclei appear pyknotic, note the relative absence of cytoplasmic shedding from small lymphocytes. From Zucker-Franklin.[138]

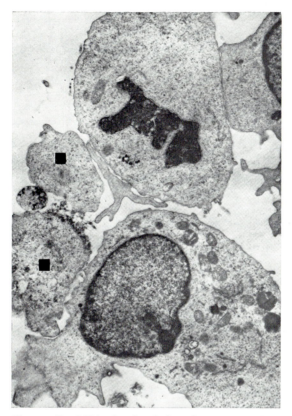

Figure 27. PHA-stimulated lymphocytes in tissue culture. Cytoplasmic droplets (square dots) to the left of the cells × 4,800. From Zucker-Franklin.[138]

cal and medullary portions in the nodes and spleen. On the other hand, in the malignant hematologic disorders, such as myeloma, lymphoma, and reticulum cell sarcoma, when hyperglobulinemia is manifest, specimens from the same organs usually show a marked increase in relative numbers of medium-sized mononuclear cells and usually cells of a single variety, e.g. plasmacytes of relatively monotonous and sometimes bizarre configuration, medium-sized lymphocytes interspersed with relatively few small lymphocytes, or huge, relatively bizarre cells resembling large lymphocytes (see Fig. 6). Although the normal-appearing mononuclear cells are seldom obliterated or totally absent, such neoplastic cells usually exceed 6 percent, 20 percent, or 10 percent of the total cell population, respectively, in the organ sampled. Sections will usually reveal obliteration of normal architecture, loss of normal relationships of cells to specific types of vessels, striking change in the corticomedullary ratio, and subtotal obliteration of elements normally expected to be present.

In the bulk of the benign and maligant hematologic disorders, such diagnostic changes may be generalized throughout the hemopoietic system but more often are localized to single clusters or kinds of hemopoietic organs. Therefore, it is often necessary to sample, as well as clinically evaluate, multiple organs to assess the true nature or extent of the disease process and to establish how much of the system is still functioning normally. Although the neoplastic or hyperplastic cells from given organs sampled may appear to shed more or less prolifically, samples from other hemopoietic organs may show normal architecture, cell-population distribution, and cytoplasmic shedding patterns.

Under these different situations, by comparing the protein composition of the blood plasma with the relative number and kind of mononuclear cells shedding cytoplasm in various hemopoietic organs, one may deduce that quantities of free extracellular proteins, especially globulins,* are being contributed to the blood. The medium-sized lymphocytes in many hemopoietic organs are relatively important contributors during health, and the plasmacytes in some hemopoietic organs become relatively important contributors during certain diseases.[97-99] Although only the contribution of plasmacytes* are recognized specifically at present, the physiologic significance of cytoplasmic shedding from each and every type of mononuclear cell may be outlined as follows.

First, owing to the fact that cytoplasm is fundamentally a gel which consists of several kinds of variably polymerized proteins, salts, and water (see Tables III and IV), the release of cellular

---

* In 1844, Donné [102] used the term "globulines" to literally describe tiny objects which he believed to be derived from lymph. The term is derived from the Latin *globulus,* meaning a tiny round object or droplet. Subsequently, the term "globulins" was used to describe free extracellular proteins soluble in weak saline solutions but differing from albumins in that they are insoluble in pure water.[59,60]

TABLE III

APPROXIMATE PERCENTAGE COMPOSITION OF
SOME MAMMALIAN TISSUES

Tissue

Component	*Striated Muscle*	*Whole Blood*	*Liver*	*Whole Brain*	*Skin*	*Bone (free of marrow)*
Water	72–78	79	60–80	78	66	20–25
Solids	22–28	21	20–40	22	34	75–80
Proteins	18–20	19	15	8	25	30
Lipids	3.0	1	3–20	12–15	7	Low
Carbohydrates	0.6	0.1	1–15	0.1	Present	Present
Organic extractives	1.0	0.14	High	1.0–2.0	Present	Low
Inorganic extractives	1.0	0.9	....	1.0	0.60	45

After E. S. West and W. R. Todd: *Textbook of Biochemistry.* New York, Macmillan, 1951.

TABLE IV

WATER CONTENT OF TISSUES

Tissue	*Water content, percent*	*Tissue*	*Water content, percent*
Brain (gray matter)	84	Liver	74
Kidneys	81	Pancreas	73
Adrenals	80	Brain (white matter)	70
Cardiac tissue	79	Skin	70
Lungs	78	Skeleton (entire)	46
Spleen	77	Adipose tissue	30‡
Brain (entire)	76	Bone (freed from marrow)	22.5
Skeletal muscle	75†	Dentine	10
Stomach and intestines	75		

* Values are approximate averages for human adult tissues.

† Skeletal muscle, comprising about 20 percent of the body weight, contains about 49 percent of the entire body water.

‡ Variable over a wide range.

After P. H. Mitchell: *A Textbook of Biochemistry.* 2d ed. New York, McGraw-Hill, 1950.

In Tables III and IV please note the relatively similar percentage distribution of water, salts, and proteins in the solid tissues (other than bone), as compared with the blood. The solid tissues and blood differ notably in how firmly water is bound to the proteins and other constituents.

cytoplasm and its dissolution (depolymerization) will result not only in the release of various free extracellular proteins but also in the release of salts and free extracellular water. Together, such free extracellular proteins, salts, and water physically constitute sols made up of proteins and salts in aqueous solution.* Upon intravascular migration, such sols constitute what we recognize as lymph or blood plasma. Thus by shedding cytoplasmic droplets, the relatively large number of mononuclear cells in various hemopoietic organs actually secrete quantities of plasma.[97]

Second, by shedding or secreting quantities of cytoplasmic water, salts, and proteins simultaneously, the various mononuclear cells create liquid media which can *flow* from the reticulum into the vascular system and *flow* onward to distant destinations, carrying various kinds of microscopically visible formed elements, along with dissolved free extracellular proteins (albumins* and globulins), salts, and other small molecules. Within the vascular system, by virtue of the colloid osmotic properties of the constituent proteins, such liquid media can retain water on the intravascular side of semipermeable membranes against the force exerted by the intravascular hydrostatic pressure under whose impetus they are impelled to flow. Thus in shedding cytoplasmic droplets and thereby secreting cytoplasmic water, salts, and proteins simultaneously, the mononuclear cells not only contribute toward the flow but also toward the maintenance of a liquid state in the blood and lymph.[97,99]

Third, shedding cytoplasm, the large and medium-sized mononuclear cells not only secrete plasma, but in doing so also lose cytoplasmic volume out of proportion to nuclear volume. In the histiocytes and macrophages, the loss of cytoplasmic volume is visibly offset by the acquisition of microscopically visible organic debris which is digested into their cytoplasm (see Fig. 5). In the plasmacytes, the loss of cytoplasmic volume appears to be offset by a relatively rapid rate of cytoplasmic growth, as reflected in cytoplasmic basophilia, pyroninophilia, ribosomal content, and well-developed endoplasmic reticulum. Relatively lacking in such

---

* Although it is not clear how much they normally secrete, it is characteristic of all plant and animal cells to synthesize albumins.

distinctive cytoplasmic features, the large and medium-sized lymphocytes continue to lose cytoplasmic volume. Thus, as they divide and differentiate, their nucleocytoplasmic ratios generally increase. Therefore, on giving rise to the small lymphocytes which constitute the bulk of the mononuclear cells to be found in the lymphoid organs, they give rise to cells relatively rich in nucleoplasm but very poor in cytoplasm. On being released with the plasma, these small cells constitute the bulk of cells in lymph, and the most common type of mononuclear cells to be found in the blood and in the tissues at large.

Chapter 10

THE DESTINY OF LYMPH

W ITH RESPECT TO its immediate destiny, the central lymph emanating from lymphoid organs flows into the arteriovenous system via central (efferent) lymphatics which join to form the paired cervical and thoracic ducts. The left thoracic duct, owing to the fact that it carries central lymph emanating from all areas below the diaphragm, is much larger than the other

Figures 28–34. All are histologically normal human tissues, surgically removed, promptly fixed in 10% neutral buffered formalin, paraffin embedded, sectioned thinly as possible, stained with hematoxylin and eosin, magnified × 1200, and photographed under oil immersion. The intraepithelial lymphocytes are marked as follows: A, Intact lymphocytes with a thin rim of cytoplasm, resembling most of the lymphocytes in the circulating blood, and within follicles of lymphoid organs. B, Intact lymphocytes as above, but with no visible cytoplasmic rim in the focal plane. C, Lymphocytes with seemingly intact nuclei but showing varying degrees of cytoplasmic swelling (presumably owing to cellular imbibition of water). D, Lymphocytes with nuclear pyknosis or chromatolysis and showing various degrees of cytoplasmic swelling. E, Lymphocytic nuclei devoid of surrounding cytoplasm, showing pyknosis or chromatolysis. F, Debris (presumably of lymphocytic origin with advanced chromatolysis and cytoplasmic degeneration) in various degrees of dispersion within the epithelium.

The total numbers of intraepithelial lymphocytes per 1000 successively encountered cells in columnar epithelia or per 1000 successively encountered basal cells in the squamous epithelia are included with each photomicrograph. In the squamous epithelia, in addition, the numbers of intraepithelial lymphocytes in the more superficial layers (per 1000 basal cells counted) are included. Of the intraepithelial lymphocytes counted in each type of endothelium, the percentages showing changes A-B, C-D, and E-F are broken down. Such differential counts represent the mean values obtained by counting approximately ten specimens of the type of epithelium under study, with each specimen being obtained from a different individual. (Although varying the depth of focal plane will reveal that many, if not most of the lymphocytes project within the cytoplasm of individual epithelial cells, the actual intracellular vs. intercellular position of the intraepithelial lymphocytes cannot be shown clearly in photomicrographs of single focal depth.)

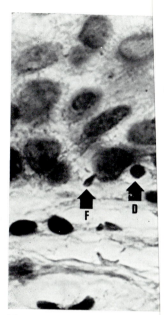

Figure 31. Cervix. Intraepithe...
1000 basal cells and 54 ± 30/...
ing ratio of basal cells: supe...
the stratified cervical epitheli...
percent.

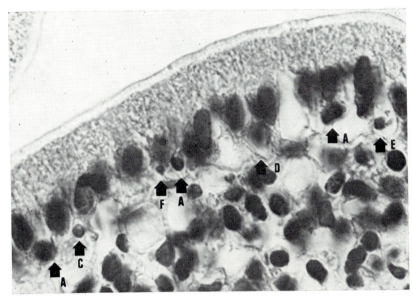

Figure 28. Jejunum. Intraepithelial lymphocytes A, C, D, E, F. Total: 75 ± 6/1000 mucosal cells. A-B 44 per cent, C-D 11 per cent, E-F 44 per cent.

kind), and are reutilized ...
Moreover, the free extra...
constituent amino acids t...
by forming linkages durin...
which carry essential me...
to their respective destinie...
sophisticated transport syst...
transported primarily via ...
testinal lymphoid tissue, ...
lymph in the thoracic du...

Second, upon being carri...
ing blood, the lymphocytes...
(e.g. 1–2 hours; see Sect...
circulation into and throug...
grate there, to be reutilized...

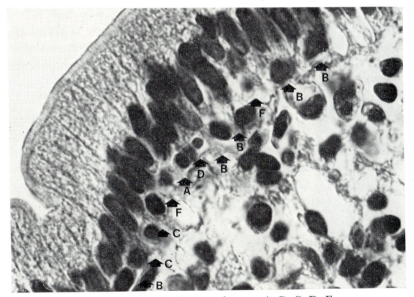

Figure 29. Jejunum. Intraepithelial lymphocytes A, B, C, D, F.

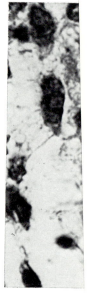

Figure 30. End
C, F. Total: 35
45 percent. Note
lymphocyte cyto

three and is g
central lymph
milky, owing
and globulins,
low concentrat
fore one must
proteins added
are removed in
destiny of lym
tissues. Such a
supported by t

First, upon
cellular protei
latter, irrespec
have been show
blood for limit

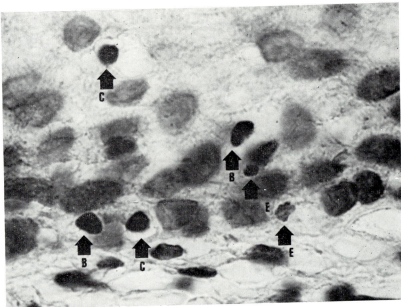

Figure 32. Cervix. Intraepithelial lymphocytes A, C, F.

illustrated in the microscopic study of the tissues under relatively high magnification, and by data obtained by isotope labeling.

Microscopic studies reveal that small lymphocyte migration, although ubiquitous, is normally quite universal not only in the interstitial layer between the small vessels and parenchymal cells of all organs,[34] but also within the parenchymal cells of those organs wherein the cell growth (or turnover) rate is relatively rapid [79-82] (see Figures 28–34). Differential counts [80,103] on small lymphocytes which have invaded parenchymal cells of various histologically normal, freshly fixed organs removed from humans are included in the legends to the figures. In the basal cells of the stratified uterine cervical epithelium, in the mucosal cells of the small intestine, in the columnar epithelial cells of the bronchi, in the endometrial mucosa cells, and in the basal epithelial cells of the cornea,* respectively, 87 ± 43, 75 ± 6, 47± 3, 35 ± 8, and

---

* Andrews [82] has differentially counted the numbers of small lymphocytes within the epidermis. The figures are not included here because it is not clear how many of the small, round cells in the skin are melanocytes. Being devoid of melanocytes, the stratified squamous epithelium of the uterine cervix and cornea were chosen for differential counting in our studies.

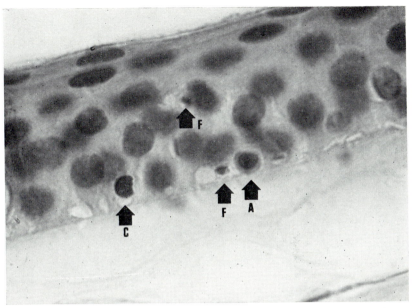

Figure 33. Cornea. Intraepithelial lymphocytes A, C, F. Total: 25 ± 10/1000 basal cells and 6 ± 4/2000 squamous cells in layers superficial (assuming ratio of basal cells/ superficial squamous cells to be 1:2) Throughout the stratified corneal epithelium A-B 15 percent, C-D 23 percent, E-F 63 percent.

25 ± 10 intracellular lymphocytes are found per 1000 of such epithelial cells successively encountered. More than one half of such intracellular (intraepithelial) lymphocytes show progressive degenerative changes including cytoplasmic swelling, nuclear pyknosis, chromatolysis, and dispersion of recognizable lymphocyte remnants within the basal cytoplasm of the epithelial cells (see Figs. 28–34).

Data obtained from isotope studies (see Chap. 16) reveal that significant quantities of labeled DNA from circulating lymphocytes are reutilized in normal small-intestinal mucosa cells,[104] and under experimental conditions (where growth is accelerated) in fibroblasts (of healing surgical wounds)[105] and in hepatic parenchymal cells (regenerating after partial hepatectomy).[106] In general, the number of small lymphocytes invading and disintegrating appears roughly proportional to the growth rate of the

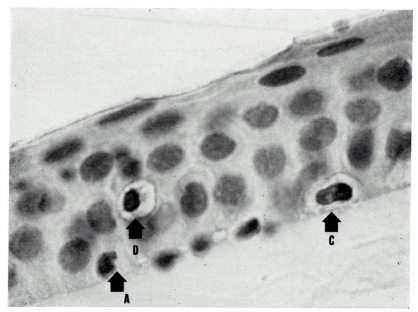

Figure 34. Cornea. Intraepithelial lymphocytes A, C, D. Note marked cytoplasmic swelling in C and D.

parenchymal cells under normal conditions and increases during the healing phase of tissue injury [1,30] (and see Chap. 16, B). In the hemopoietic organs and particularly the lymphoid organs, wherein the cellular growth rate appears exceedingly rapid as compared with that of parenchymal cells in other organs, relatively large numbers of small lymphocytes are found disintegrating, especially within histiocytes and macrophages, as shown by Kindred.[9-11]

Such microscopic and supplementary isotopic findings indicate that the small lymphocytes not only migrate into other kinds of cells but also that they visibly feed the latter by donating their substance (particularly their nucleoplasm containing DNA). The immunologic as well as trophic significance of these findings, with special reference to lymphocyte migration and disintegration in lymphoid organs, will be discussed in greater detail later.

Chapter 11

DISCUSSION

A T PRESENT, IT IS generally agreed [7,8] that the lymphoid organs have three definitive functions, each of immunologic import:

1. To filter and remove foreign proteins from the blood and lymph—a function performed by histiocytes and macrophages in the spleen and lymph nodes (as well as in the marrow, liver, and loose connective tissues) .[44,54]
2. To produce specific free extracellular proteins, called antibodies, immune globulins, or immunoglobulins, which agglutinate or precipitate foreign proteins, thus hastening their phagocytosis in histiocytes and macrophages; or which opsonize (Greek translation, "prepare as food") bacteria to facilitate their ingestion into macrophages and microphages (polymorphonuclear leucocytes) .
3. To produce small lymphocytes which lyse foreign cells directly (see Chap. 16, B) , and which seem to transform into plasmacytes (see Chap. 16, B) .

With respect to the first function, it remains to be settled how and in what form the histiocytes and macrophages dispose of the foreign proteins they ingest and digest into their cytoplasm.

With respect to the second function (as already mentioned) , it remains to be settled how and in what form the plasmacytes secrete immunoglobulins from their cytoplasm; whether they are the sole source of immunoglobulins; how the immunoglobulins, known to be of relatively short biologic life, are replicated and replaced continually during health, as well as during various disease processes; and how they are broken down and reutilized under both circumstances. Although it is fundamental that when cells synthesize proteins and grow, they also take in water and salts which are variably bound to their proteins, review of the current literature on plasmacytes will reveal that few consider finitive kind of mononuclear cell by Ramon y Cajal [122] and by Unna.[123] Their descriptions differed, with Unna maintaining that deep cytoplasmic basophilia and pyroninophilia were the most distinctive features, along with a slightly spongy appearance of the cytoplasm; whereas Cajal considered their differentiation without karyokinesis (mitosis) to be an additional distinctive feature. In 1895, von Marschalkó [124] stressed that in addition to great cytoplasmic affinity for basic stains, the following criteria were essential in identifying plasmacytes:

1. A cartwheel-like blocking of chromatin in the nucleus.

2. An eccentric position of the nucleus.

3. A paranuclear pale staining halo.

4. Lack of specific granules in the cytoplasm.

As the years passed, some continued to use Unna's definition, whereas others adhered to the additional criteria imposed by von Marschalkó. Several, such as Downey,[36,101] Weidenreich,[36,87,88] Maximow,[35,47] and Michels,[125] pointed out that large lymphocytes, as they differentiate, pass through a deeply basophilic, pyroninophilic stage wherein they cannot be differentiated morphologically from Unna's plasmacytes. In general, German and north European histologists have continued to define the plasmacyte in the manner of Unna, while Latin and some American hematologists have adhered to von Marschalkó's criteria. Weidenreich [36,87,88] concluded that all the deeply basophilic mononuclear cells were secretory corpuscles, whether or not they ultimately developed into typical von Marschalkó-type plasmacytes or into lymphocytes. As already mentioned, he pointed to their cytoplasmic shedding as evidence of a secretory function, but did not define the secretory product. In 1922, de Assua [126] emphasized the degenerative changes in plasmacytes as well as their cytoplasmic shedding as evidence for their secretory function. More recently, Ehrich [119] reemphasized that under normal conditions, the plasmacytes disintegrate within the hemopoietic organs (instead of emigrating like lymphocytes). With the application of spectrophotometry to the study of cells, Brachet [127] stressed that the deep cytoplasmic basophilia of plasmacytes and many of the lymphocytes is owing to a high cytoplasmic concentration of RNA, and is a sign of relatively active intracytoplasmic protein synthesis. Under the electron microscope, the latter capacity is reflected in the development of ribosomes and a coarse endoplasmic reticulum [34] which, incidentally, is probably responsible for the spongy appearance of plasmacyte cytoplasm as it was described by Unna.

Although it is not recognized currently that the plasmacytes secrete plasma, it is generally recognized that during the early stages of the immunologic reaction to foreign proteins [90-94] (see Chap. 18) and in certain diseases such as myeloma [95,128] (plasma cell tumor in bone), the plasmacytes secrete a variety of free extracellular proteins which precipitate or agglutinate known antigens. Such proteins, known as immunoglobulins, as already mentioned, constitute some 5 to 10 percent of the plasma proteins.[73-77] On the basis of their capacity to agglutinate other proteins, Coons and Leduc,[129] by labeling globulins produced in sensitized rabbits with fluorescent dyes, definitively traced the origin of immunoglobulins to plasmacytes during the second to sixth day of the primary immunologic response. These data, together with the aforementioned observations on cytoplasmic basophilia, pyroninophilia, endoplasmic reticulum in plasmacytes, and their relative numerical increase in diseases wherein serum globulin concentrations are relatively increased, have led to the currently popular conclusion that the plasmacytes secrete the bulk of immunoglobulins to be found in the blood.[59,60,73-77,128]

With respect to the precise nature of free extracellular proteins produced by plasmacytes, the subject remains under intensive clinical and experimental study. Thus far, it has become apparent that they are capable of producing a wide variety of globulins of differing molecular weight, electrophoretic mobility, and immunoelectrophoretic pattern.[73,128] Many of these differ from remaining normal serum globulins only in their terminal or prosthetic molecular groups.[130] It seems significant that in the clinical studies wherein a marked increase in certain specific globulins are found, the majority of the plasmacytes apparently responsible prove to be of a relatively immature variety, and a variety not seen in great numbers in lymphoid tissues or bone marrow under normal conditions.[91,92,128] Of significance to note with relatively high-molecular-weight, electrophoretically slow-moving nucleoproteins. Thus, both the quantities and qualities of plasma the lymphocytes produce by cytoplasmic shedding must remain open to question.

Looking toward the nuclear material, evidence has been presented to indicate that the small lymphocytes, depleted of cytoplasm by shedding from their larger precursors, may supplement the nutritive function of the latter by emigrating from the lym-

TABLE V

ELECTROPHORETIC COMPARISON OF THE FREE EXTRACELLULAR PROTEINS IN THE SERUM OF A PATIENT HAVING CHRONIC LYMPHO-CYTIC LEUKEMIA* WITH THE FREE EXTRACELLULAR PROTEINS OBTAINED BY SAPONIN LYSIS OF HIS SALINE-WASHED LYMPHOCYTES

	Serum %	Leukemic Lymphocytes %
Albumin	64.5	4.1
Alpha$_1$ globulin	2.6	11.5
Alpha$_2$ globulin	6.8	16.0
Beta globulin	14.8	20.0
Gamma globulin	12.0	48.4

* W.B.C., 600,000.

phoid organs in the plasma to carry their nucleoplasm actively to cells in other kinds of tissues, especially some of the rapidly growing epithelia. In so doing, the small lymphocytes may transport relatively large molecules of great biologic significance,[109,110] whose penetration into the tissues would be very slow by the process of simple diffusion (owing to relatively high molecular weight). Although the mechanisms of their reutilization are not obvious, it seems clear that the large precursors of lymphocytes, through shedding plasma, and the small lymphocytes, by migrating passively in the plasma and then actively through the tissues, must perform trophic functions there as disintegration proceeds.

With respect to their simultaneous immunologic functions, the lymphocytes remain under intensive clinical and experimental study. Thus far, it has become apparent that upon appropriate sensitization—a process involving multiple kinds of mononuclear cells (see Chaps. 18 and 24, C)—significant numbers of small circulating lymphocytes become capable of lysing cells from a genetically incompatible donor and sometimes the body's own cells.[78] In so doing, the small lymphocytes may not only destroy living matter which is genetically incompatible, spurious, or foreign but also reduce the latter by lysis into forms of substrate reutilizable in the histiocytes, macrophages, and other cells in the individual. Moreover, as it has been found that immunologic memory resides within small lymphocytes, particularly in their nuclear DNA, it would appear they remain capable of performing such simultaneous immunologic and trophic functions for extended periods of time. It remains, therefore, to ascertain whether such simultaneous functions are best served by a population of small lymphocytes of prolonged biological life or by a short-lived population whose nuclear DNA has an inherent plasticity, as well as stability (see Chap. 18, B).

Although White and Dougherty [20-23] did not suggest that lymphocytes secrete quantities of plasma, pursuant to their studies on the biochemical composition of lymphoid cells and their propensity to shed cytoplasm and undergo lysis at accelerated rates with adrenal glucocorticoid stimulation, they concluded that lymphocytes (size unspecified) normally synthesize and secrete normal globulins, as well as immune globulins. Like Sabin's earlier conclusion that antigen-stimulated macrophages secrete antibodies along with other free extracellular proteins by cytoplasmic shedding, White and Dougherty's conclusions were overshadowed and not generally accepted, because almost simultaneously published experimental and clinical observations indicated that plasmacytes are the source of immunoglobulins (see above), whereas liver cells appear to be the source of remaining plasma proteins (see Sect. 3).

5. Functional Semantics

Thus, from a functional, as well as morphologic point of view it has become apparent that the various kinds of mononuclear cells are endowed either with definitions which are imprecise, or with multiple, overlapping functions, as in the following examples.

The term "plasmablasts" literally means precursors of plasma, but the term is now generally used to describe the large, immature precursors of plasmacytes. Fagraeus[92] has emphasized that the relatively large plasmablasts, not the smaller plasmacytes, appear to be the principal source of immunoglobulins during the early stages of the immune response and in myelomas—as well as being the precursors of smaller plasmacytes.

The term "lymphoblasts" literally means precursors of lymph, but the term is now generally used to describe the larger, immature precursors of small lymphocytes. As lymph consists of plasma as well as cells (mostly small lymphocytes), it is problematic whether this term should be used in the broad sense to describe the precursors of lymph or in a narrower sense to describe the precursors of small lymphocytes. For this reason, the use of this term is avoided in the text; the terms "large," "medium-sized," and "small" lymphocytes are more specific, at least from a morphologic point of view.

As already mentioned, the term "clasmatocytes" literally means fragment cells, but the term is no longer used generally. Instead, the term "macrophages" (big eaters) is commonly used to describe the same cells. It is problematic whether the shedding of cytoplasmic fragments or the ingestion of microscopically visible particulate matter is the most important aspect of such cells. Moreover, as various kinds of nonphagocytic mononuclear cells (such as plasmacytes and lymphocytes) appear to shed cytoplasmic fragments also, it is problematic whether all or some specific ones should be called clasmatocytes.

Relatively recently, in order to avoid the use of imprecise or confusing morphologic terms, the terms "immunoblasts" (precursors of immunity) and "immunocytes" (immune cells) have come into popular usage to describe plasmacytes and lymphocytes in terms of function.[134] Such terms may be quite apropos if their only function is immunologic. But if their function is also nutritive, the terms "trophoblasts" (precursors of food), "trophocytes" (food cells), or "trephocytes" (feeding cells; see Sect. 2) might be just as good. Recognizing that such cells may be polyfunctional, one might compound terms, such as immune (sensitized) trephocytes or nonimmune (nonsensitized) trephocytes to indicate functions seeming most important at a given time. Another alternative is to continue use of time-worn morphologic descriptions, such as mononuclear cells (one nucleus cells), lymphoid cells (cells like lymphocytes), or lymphoid elements (elements related to lymph) to describe the elements collectively, without singling out any particular function. Finally, with the clear implication that the functions of lymphoid elements (including lymphoid organs, mononuclear cells, lymph, and plasma) are *trophic,* as well as *immunologic,* in order to describe how the former are interrelated, one may choose to continue to use the old terms, such as "plasmablasts" (precursors of plasma), "lymphoblasts" (precursors of lymph), "plasmacytes" (plasma cells), and "lymphocytes" (lymph cells), with a fuller meaning!

Chapter 12

SUMMARY

DATA FROM THE literature and a series of previously published personal observations are reviewed and correlated to indicate that the normal function of lymphoid organs is to mediate the transport of nourishment to other tissues. The data is organized to indicate that they do this by converting molecules from their afferent arteries, from the mucosal cells lining the gut, and from peripheral lymphatics into rapidly growing mononuclear cell populations which normally constitute 1 to 2 percent of total body weight. These mononuclear cell populations, in turn, give rise to lymph consisting of plasma and free cells (mostly small lymphocytes). Histologic evidence is presented to show that the plasma arises by dissolution of cytoplasmic droplets shed from several kinds of relatively large mononuclear cells in the lymphoid organs, whereas the small, cytoplasm-poor lymphocytes develop through loss of such cytoplasmic droplets from their larger, dividing precursors. The plasma, in turn, carries water, salts, various kinds of small molecules, and several kinds of free extracellular proteins (especially globulins) to be reutilized in other tissues. The small, cytoplasm-poor lymphocytes, being independently motile and invasive cells, actively transport relatively large molecules, such as nucleoproteins, to be reutilized there when they disintegrate.

On the basis of their characteristic vascular supply and relation to other tissues, the trophic or feeding function of various kinds of lymphoid tissue are tentatively outlined, with the intestinal lymphoid tissue being concerned primarily with the active internal transport of newly absorbed proteins and fats, the spleen being concerned with the storage of proteins to buffer the loss of proteins from the intestinal lymphoid tissue between meals and during starvation, the nodes being concerned with the processing and reutilization of proteins which emanate from the peripheral tissues, the thymus and the periarteriolar lymphoid tissue of the marrow having trophic functions to be considered in some detail in ensuing sections of this book.

On the basis of their distinctive characteristic features, the trophic function of various kinds of mononuclear cells are tentatively outlined; the reticular cells are concerned with a matrical function in support of the blood and lymph elements, as well as the parenchymal cells in peripheral tissues; the histiocytes and macrophages are involved with the ingestion and digestion of endogenous and exogenous proteins which, by shedding cytoplasm, they release to be reutilized elsewhere; the plasmacytes are involved with the formation of plasma, including many of its immunoglobulins; the larger lymphocytes are also involved with the formation of plasma, especially its normal globulins; and the smaller lymphocytes are involved with the transport of nucleoproteins by active migration into the tissues.

Moreover, the data is organized to indicate that simultaneously, by reutilizing foreign proteins brought in via the same afferent pathways, the lymphoid organs may produce modified globulins (immunoglobulins) and modified (immunologically competent) small lymphocytes which augment the normal trophic function of the lymphoid tissues by destroying foreign proteins and their living sources, so that both of the latter may be reutilized for food in various kinds of cells in the host.

REFERENCES

1. Rich, A. R.: Inflammation in resistance to infection. *Arch Path, 22:* 228–254, 1936.

2. Trowell, O. A.: The lymphocyte. *Int. Rev Cytol, 7:*236–293, 1958.

3. Shields, J. W.: *An Evaluation of Splenic Puncture as a Procedure in the Diagnosis of Hematologic Disorders.* Mayo Foundation Thesis, 1956.

4. Maximow, A.: Relation of blood cells to connective tissues and endothelium. *Physiol Rev, 4:*533–563, 1924.

5. Maximow, A.: Morphology of the mesenchymal reactions. *Arch Path Lab Med, 4:*557–606, 1927.

6. Wintrobe, M. M.: *Clinical Hematology,* 6th ed. Philadelphia, Lea & Febiger, 1967.

7. Drinker, C. K. and Yoffey, J. M.: *Lymphatics, Lymph, and Lymphoid Tissue.* Cambridge, Harvard University Press, 1941.

8. Yoffey, J. M. and Courtice, F. C.: *Lymphatics, Lymph, and Lymphoid Tissue.* Cambridge, Harvard University Press, 1956.

9. Kindred, J. E.: Quantitative studies on lymphoid tissues. *Ann NY Acad Sci, 59:*746–756, 1955.

10. Kindred, J. E.: A quantitative study of the haemopoietic organs of young albino rats. *Amer J Anat, 67:*99–149, 1940.

11. Kindred, J. E.: A quantitative study of the haemopoietic organs of young adult albino rats. *Amer J Anat, 71:*207–243, 1942.

12. Yoffey, J. M.: Further problems of lymphocyte production. *Ann NY Acad Sci, 113:*867–886, 1964.

13. Leblond, C. P. and Walker, B. E.: Renewal of cell populations. *Physiol Rev, 36:*255–276, 1956.

14. Perry, S., Craddock, C. G., Ventzke, L., Crepaldi, G., and Lawrence, J. S.: Rate of production of ^{32}P labeled lymphocytes. *Blood, 14:* 50–59, 1959.

15. Bloom, W.: *Histopathology of Irradiation from External and Internal Sources.* New York, McGraw-Hill, 1948.

16. Errera, M.: Biochime et Radiobiologie du Noyau Cellulaire. In Harris, R. J. C. (Ed.) : *The Initial Effects of Ionizing Radiations on Cells.* New York, Academic Press, 1961, pp. 165–172.

17. Stocken, L. A.: Phosphate metabolism in the nucleus. In Harris, R. J. C. (Ed.) : *The Initial Effects of Ionizing Radiations on Cells.* New York, Academic Press, 1961, pp. 195–200.

18. Pollard, E.: The action of ionizing radiation on the cellular synthesis of protein. In Harris, R. J. C. (Ed.) : *The Initial Effects of Ionizing Radiations on Cells.* New York, Academic Press, 1961, pp. 75–90.

19. Loutit, J. F.: Immunologic and trophic functions of lymphocytes. *Lancet, 2:*1106–1108, 1962.

20. Dougherty, T. F. and White, A.: Effect of pituitary adrenotrophic hormone on lymphocytes. *Proc Soc Exp Biol Med, 53:*132–133, 1943.

21. White, A. and Dougherty, T. F.: The role of lymphocytes in normal and immune globulin production and the mode of release of globulin from lymphocytes. *Ann NY Acad Sci, 46:*859–882, 1946.

22. White, A.: Effects of steroids on aspects of the metabolism and functions of the lymphocyte: A hypothesis of the cellular mechanisms in antibody formation and related immune phenomena. *Ann NY Acad Sci, 73:*79–104, 1958.

23. White, A.: Influence of endocrine secretions on the structure and function of lymphoid tissue. In *Harvey Lectures.* Springfield, Thomas, 1950, pp. 43–70.

24. Selye, H.: *The Physiology and Pathology of Exposure to Stress.* Montreal, Acta, 1950.

25. Ivy, A. C.: Gastrointestinal changes in the rat on realimentation. *Amer J Physiol, 195:*216–220, 1958.

26. MacKenzie, D. W., Whipple, A. O., and Wintersteiner, M. P.: Studies on microscopic anatomy and physiology of living transilluminated mammalian spleens. *Amer J Anat, 68:*397–456, 1941.

27. Hofmeister, F.: Untersuchungen über Resorption und Assimilation der Nährstoffe. *Arch Exp Path Pharmkol, 19:*1–83, 1885.

28. Hammar, J. A.: Zur Histogenese und Involution der Thymusdruese. *Anat Anz, 27:*23, 41, 1905.

29. Hammar, J. A.: *Die normal-morphologische Thymusforschung.* Leipzig, J. A. Barth, 1936.

30. Boyd, W.: *A Textbook of Pathology.* Philadelphia, Lea & Febiger, 1961.

31. Dameshek, W.: William Hewson, thymicologist; father of hematology? *Blood, 21:*513–516, 1963.

32. Dustin, A. P.: Recherches d'histologie normale, et experimentale sur le thymus des amphibious anoures. *Arch Biol (Liege), 28:*1, 1913.

33. Dustin, A. P. and Gregoire, C.: Contribution a l'étude de la mitose diminutive au elassatique dans le thymus des mammiferes. *C. R. Soc. Biol. (Paris), 108:*1, 159, 1931.

34. Bloom, W. and Fawcett, D. W.: *Textbook of Histology.* Philadelphia, Saunders, 1968, pp. 1–21.

35. Bloom, W.: Lymphatic Tissue, Lymphatic Organs. In Downey, H. (Ed.) : *Handbook of Hematology.* New York, Hoeber, 1938, vol. 2, pp. 1427–1468.

36. Downey, H. and Weidenreich, F.: Ueber die Bildung der Lymphocyten in lymphdruesen und Milz. *Arch Mikr Anat, 80*:306–395, 1912.

37. Möllendorf, W. and Möllendorf, M.: Das Fibrocytennetz im lockeren Bindegewebe; sein wandlungsfähigkeit und anteilnahme am stoffwechsel. *Z Zellforsch, 3*:503–614, 1926.

38. Cunningham, R. S., Sabin, F. R., and Doan, C. A.: The development of leucocytes, lymphocytes, and monocytes from a specific stem cell in adult tissues. *Contrib. to Embryol. #84, Carnegie Inst. Wash., 16*: 227–276, 1925.

39. Danchakoff, V.: Equivalence of different hematopoietic anlages. *Amer J Anat, 24*:127–189, 1918.

40. Klemperer, P.: The relationship of the Reticulum to Diseases of the Hematopoietic System. In *Contribution to the Medical Sciences in Honor of Dr. Emanuel Libman by his Pupils, Friends, and Colleagues.* New York, International Press, 1932, pp. 655–672.

41. Klemperer, P.: The spleen. In Downey, H. (Ed.) : *Handbook of Hematology.* New York, Hoeber, 1938, vol. 3, pp. 1587–1754.

42. Bessis, M.: *Cytology of the Blood and Blood-Forming Organs.* New York, Grune and Stratton, 1956.

43. Aschoff, L.: Das reticulo-endotheliale system. *Ergebn Inn Med Kinderheilk, 26*:1–119, 1924. (Also in *Lectures on Pathology,* New York, Hoeber, 1924, pp. 1–33.)

44. Downey, H.: The structure and origin of the lymph sinuses of mammalian lymph nodes and their relations to endothelium and reticulum. *Hematology, 3*:431–468, 1922.

45. Isaacs, R.: The physiologic histology of bone marrow: The mechanism of the development of blood cells and their liberation into the peripheral circulation. *Folia Haemat, 40*:395–405, 1930.

46. Bloom, W.: Fibroblasts and macrophages (histiocytes) . In Downey, H. (Ed.) : *Handbook of Hematology.* New York, Hoeber, 1938, pp. 1335–1373.

47. Bloom, W.: Lymphocytes and monocytes: Theories of hematopoiesis. In Downey, H. (Ed.) : *Handbook of Hematology.* New York, Hoeber, 1938, pp. 375–435 and 1551–1585.

48. Bloom, W.: Embryogenesis of mammalian blood. In Downey, H. (Ed.) : *Handbook of Hematology.* New York, Hoeber, 1938, pp. 862–922.

49. Jordan, H. E.: Comparative hematology. In Downey, H. (Ed.) : *Handbook of Hematology.* New York, Hoeber, 1938, pp. 699–862.

50. Bloom, W.: Myelopoietic potency of fixed cells of the rabbit liver. *Libmann Anniv Vols (II),* 1932, pp. 199–207.

51. Mann, J. D. and Higgins, C. M.: The system of fixed histiocytes in the liver. In Downey, H. (Ed.) : *Handbook of Hematology.* New York, Hoeber, 1938, pp. 1370–1426.

52. Sabin, F. R.: Bone marrow. In Cowdry, E. V. (Ed.) : *Special Cytology.* New York, Hoeber, 1932, pp. 507–527.

53. Shields, J. W.: On the relationship between growing blood cells and blood vessels. *Acta Haemat (Basel), 24*:319–329, 1960.

54. Jaffé, R. H.: The reticulo-endothelial system. In Downey, H. (Ed.) : *Handbook of Hematology.* New York, Hoeber, 1938, pp. 977–1271.

55. Ranvier, L.: Des Clamatocytes. *Compt Rend Acad Sci, 110*:165–169, 1890.

56. Metchnikoff, E.: *Immunity in Infective Diseases.* (English ed. by F. G. Binnie) , Cambridge, Cambridge University Press, 1905.

57. Doan, C. A.: Bone marrow. Normal and pathologic physiology with special reference to diseases involving the cells of the blood. In Downey, H. (Ed.) : *Handbook of Hematology.* New York, Hoeber, 1938, pp. 1839–1962.

58. Michels, N. A.: The mast cells. In Downey, H. (Ed.) : *Handbook of Hematology.* New York, Hoeber, 1938, pp. 231–372.

59. Best, C. H. and Taylor, N. B.: *The Physiological Basis of Medical Practice,* 5th ed. Baltimore, Williams & Wilkins, 1966.

60. White, A., Handler, P., Smith, E. L., and Stetten, D.: *Principles of Biochemistry,* 4th ed. Toronto, McGraw-Hill, 1968.

61. Ehrich, W. E.: The role of the lymphocytes in the circulation of lymph. *Ann NY Acad Sci, 46*:823–857, 1946.

62. Grant, J. L. and Smith, B.: Bone marrow gas tensions, bone marrow blood flow and erythropoiesis in man. *Ann Intern Med, 58*:801–809, 1963.

63. Trowell, O. A.: Experiments on lymph nodes cultured *in vitro. Ann NY Acad Sci, 59*:1066–1069, 1955.

64. Moeschlin, S.: *Spleen Puncture.* London, Heinemann, 1951.

65. Forkner, C. E.: Material from lymph nodes of man. I. Method to obtain material by puncture of lymph nodes for study with supravital and fixed stains. II. Studies on living and fixed cells withdrawn from lymph nodes of man. *Arch Intern Med,* (I) *40*:532–537; (II) 647–660, 1927.

66. Tempka, T. and Kubiczek, M.: Normal and pathologic lymphadenogram in light of own research. *Acta Med Scand, 131*:434–450, 1948.

67. André, R. and Dreyfuss, B.: La Ponction Ganglionaire. In *Langres, Exposition Scientifique Francaise,* 1954.

68. Shields, J. W. and Hargraves, M. M.: An evaluation of splenic puncture. *Proc Staff Meet Mayo Clin, 31*:440–453, 1956.

69. Witte, C. L., Clauss, R. H., and Dumont, A. E.: Respiratory gas tensions of thoracic duct lymph. An index of gas exchange in splanchnic tissues. *Ann Surg, 166*:254–262, 1967.

70. Bierman, H. R., Byron, R. L., Kelley, K. H., Gilfillan, R. S., White, L., Freeman, N. E., and Petrakis, N.: The characteristics of thoracic duct lymph in man. *J Clin Invest., 32*:637–649, July, 1953.

71. Bierman, H. R., Kelly, K. H., White, L. P., Coblentz, A., and Fisher, A.: Transhepatic venous catheterization and venography. *JAMA, 158*: 1331, 1955.

72. Whipple, G. H.: *The Dynamic Equilibrium of Body Proteins.* Springfield, Thomas, 1956.

73. Mannik, M. and Kunkel, H. G.: The immunoglobulins. In Samter, M. and Alexander, H. L. (Eds.) : *Immunological Diseases.* Boston, Little, Brown, 1965, pp. 278–304.

74. Miller, L. L., Bly, C. G., Watson, M. L., and Bale, W. F.: The dominant role of the liver in plasma protein synthesis. A direct study of isolated perfused rat liver with the aid of lysine with C-14. *J Exp Med, 94*:431–453, 1951.

75. Miller, L. L. and Bale, W. F.: Synthesis of all plasma protein fractions except gamma globulins by the liver. The use of zone electrophoresis and lysine with C-14 to define the proteins synthesized by the isolated perfused liver. *J Exp Med, 99*:125–132, 1954.

76. Miller, L. L., Bly, C. G., and Bale, W. F.: Plasma and tissue proteins produced by non-hepatic rat organs as studied with lysine C-14. Gamma globulins the chief plasma protein fraction produced by non-hepatic tissue. *J Exp Med, 99*:133–153, 1954.

77. Simmons, P., Penny, R., and Goller, I.: Plasma proteins: A review. *Med J Aust, 2*:494–506, 1969.

78. Sherwin, R. P.: *The Embattled Cell.* A movie sponsored by the American Cancer Society, 1967.

79. Humble, J. G., Jayne, W. H. W., and Pulvertaft, R. J. V.: Biological interaction between lymphocytes and other cells. *Brit J Haemat, 2*:283–294, 1956.

80. Shields, J. W., Touchon, R. C., and Dickson, D. R.: Quantitative studies on small lymphocyte disposition in epithelial cells. *Amer J Path, 54*:129–145, 1969.

81. Schaffer, J.: Leucocyten im Epithel. In Moellendorf, W. V. (Ed.) : *Handbuch der Mikr Anat,* 1927.

82. Andrew, W. and Andrew, N. V.: Lymphocytes in the normal epidermis of the rat and of man. *Anat Rec, 104*:217–241, 1949.

83. Dominici, M.: Histologie de la rate normale. *Arch Med Exp Anat Path, 12*:563–588, 1900.

84. Dominici, M.: Histologie de la rate au cours des états infectieux. *Arch Med Exp Anat Path, 12*:733–768, 1900.

85. Wright, J. H.: The histiogenesis of the blood platelets. *J Morph, 21*:263–278, 1910.

86. Downey, H.: The origin of blood platelets. *Folia Haemat, 1*:25–58, 1913.

87. Weidenreich, R.: Zur Morphologie und morphologischen Stellung der ungranulierten Leucocytes - Lymphocyten des Blutes und der Lymphe. *Arch Mikr Anat, 73*:793, 1909.

88. Weidenreich, F.: Die Leucocyten und verwadte Zellformen. *Ergebn Anat Entwicklungsgesch, 19*:527, 1911.

89. Sabin, F. R.: Cellular reactions to a dye-protein with a concept of the mechanism of antibody formation. *J Exp Med, 70*:67–82, 1939.

90. McMaster, P. D. and Hudack, S. S.: The formation of agglutinins within lymph nodes. *J. Exp Med, 61*:783–805, 1935,

91. Bjørneboe, M. and Gormsen, H.: Experimental studies on the role of plasma cells as antibody producers. *Acta Pathol Microbiol Scand, 20*:649–691, 1943.

92. Fagraeus, A.: Antibody production in relation to the development of plasma cells. *Acta Med Scand, 130* (suppl. 204) :3–122, 1948.

93. Ehrich, W. E., Drabkin, D. L., and Furman, C.: Nucleic acids and the production of antibody by plasma cells. *J Exp Med, 90*:157–168, 1949.

94. Harris, T. N. and Harris, S.: Histochemical changes in lymphocytes during production of antibodies in lymph nodes of rabbits. *J Exp Med, 90*:169–180, 1949.

95. Leitner, S. J.: *Bone Marrow Biopsy. Hematology in the Light of Sternal Puncture.* (English ed. by Britton, C.J.C. and Neumark, E.) New York, Grune & Stratton, 1949.

96. Engelbert, V. E.: Cells of the thymus and their release of cytoplasmic portions *in vitro. Canad J Zool, 31*:106–111, 1953.

97. Shields, J. W.: Mononuclear cells, hyaline bodies, and the plasma. An analytic review. *Blood, 17*:235–251, 1961.

98. Shields, J. W.: On the function of lymphoid tissue. *Proceedings of the IX Congress of the International Society of Hematology, 3*:621–629, 1964.

99. Shields, J. W.: Hypothesis on the role of the reticulum and lymphoid tissues in water and food transport. *Blood, 27*:883–894, 1966.

100. Rondanelli, E. G., Magliola, G., Carosi, G., and Dionosi, D.: Cytoplasmic shedding as a mode of formation of lymphocyte-like blast cells by newt histiocytes. *Acta Haemat, 40*:67–74, 1968.

101. Downey, H.: The origin and structure of the plasma cells of normal vertebrates, and the eosinophils of the lung of ambylostoma. *Folia Haemat, 11*:257, 1911.

102. Donné, A.: *Cours de Microscopie.* Paris, Bailliere, 1844.

103. Van Buskirk, M. and Shields, J. W.: Personal observations.

104. Fichtelius, K. E. and Bryant, B. J.: On the fate of thymocytes. In Good, R. A. and Gabrielson, A. E. (Eds.) : *The Thymus in Immunobiology.* New York, Hoeber, 1964, pp. 274–287.

105. Fichtelius, K. E. and Diderholm, H.: Autoradiographic analysis of the accumulation of lymphocytes in wounds. *Acta Path Microbiol Scand, 52*:11–18, 1961.

106. Bryant, B. J.: Reutilization of leukocyte DNA by cells of regenerating liver. *Exp Cell Res, 27*:70–79, 1962.

107. Wiseman, B. K.: The identity of the lymphocyte. *Folia Haemat, 46*:346–358, 1932.
108. Elves, M. W.: *The Lymphocytes.* Chicago, Year Book Medical Publishers, 1967.
109. Kelsall, M. A. and Crabb, E. D.: Lymphocytes and plasmacytes and nucleoprotein metabolism. *Ann NY Acad Sci, 72*:293–337, 1958.
110. Kelsall, M. A. and Crabb, E. D.: *Lymphocytes and Mast Cells.* Baltimore, Williams & Wilkins, 1959.
111. Shields, J. W.: Intestinal lymphoid tissue activity during absorption. *Amer J Gastroent, 50*:30–36, 1968.
112. Brandborg, L. L.: The lamina propria: orphan of the gut. *Gastroenterology, 57*:191–193, 1969.
113. Halliday, R.: The absorption of antibodies from immune sera by the gut of the young rat. *Proc Roy Soc (Biol), 143*:408–413, 1955.
114. Brambell, F. W. R.: The passive immunity of the young mammal. *Biol Rev, 33*:488–531, 1958.
115. Crosby, W. H.: Normal functions of the spleen relative to red blood cells. *Blood, 14*:399–408, 1959.
116. Wiseman, B. K. and Doan, C. A.: Primary splenic neutropenia; a newly recognized syndrome, closely related to congenital hemolytic icterus of essential thrombocytopenic purpura. *Ann Int Med, 16*:1097–1117, 1942.
117. Dameshek, W. and Estren, S.: *The Spleen and Hypersplenism.* New York, Grune & Stratton, 1947.
118. Fitch, F. W. and Wissler, R. W.: The histology of antibody production. In Samter, M. and Alexander, H. L. (Eds.): *Immunological Diseases.* Boston, Little, Brown, 1965, pp. 65–86.
119. Ehrich, W. E.: Lymphoid tissues: Their morphology and role in the immune response. In Samter, M. and Alexander, H. L. (Eds.): *Immunological Diseases.* Boston, Little, Brown, 1965, pp. 250–277.
120. Fishman, M.: Antibody formation in vitro. *J Exp Med, 114*:837–856, 1961.
121. Waldeyer, W.: Ueber Bindegewebzellen. *Arch Mikr Anat, 11*:176, 1875.
122. Ramon y Cajal: *Manual de anatomia patologica general,* ed. 1. Barcelona, 1890.
123. Unna, P.: Ueber Plasmazellen, insbesondere beim Lupus. *Monatschr Prakt Dermat, 12*:296–317, 1891.
124. von Marschalkó, T.: Ueber die soganannten Plasmazellen: Ein Beitrag zur Kenntnis der Herkunft der entzundlichen Infiltrationzellen. *Arch Derm Syph, 30*:3, 1895; *30*:241, 1895.
125. Michels, N. A. L.: The plasma cell: A critical review of its morphogenesis, function and developmental capacity under normal and under abnormal conditions. *Arch Path, 11*:775–793, 1931.

126. de Assua, Jiminez: Células cianófilas y celulas cebadas. *Arch Cardiol Hemat, 3*:1, 1922.

127. Brachet, J.: The localization and the role of ribonucleic acid in the cell. *Ann NY Acad Sci, 50*:861–869, 1950.

128. Levin, W. C. and Ritzmann, S. E.: Relation of abnormal proteins to formed elements of the blood: Cellular sources. *Ann Rev Med, 16*:187–200, 1965.

129. Coons, A. H., Leduc, E. H., and Connolly, J. M.: Studies on antibody production: I. A method for the histochemical demonstration of specific antibody and its application to a study of the hyperimmune rabbit. *J Exp Med, 102*:49–60, 1955.

130. Nisonoff, A.: Molecules of immunity. *Hosp Pract, 2* (6) :19–27, 1967.

131. Stenzel, K. H. and Rubin, A. L.: Biosynthesis of gamma globulin: Studies in a cell-free system. *Science, 153*:537–539, 1966.

132. Good, R. A. and Varco, R. L.: A clinical and experimental study on agammaglobulinemia. In *Essays on Pediatrics.* Minneapolis, Lancet, 1955, pp. 103–129.

133. Samter, M., Ed.: *Immunological Diseases.* Boston, Little, Brown, 1965.

134. Dameshek, W.: "Immunocytes" and "immunoblasts"—An attempt at a functional nomenclature. *Blood, 21*:243–245, 1963.

135. Goodman, J. R. and Hall, S. G.: Plasma cells containing iron: An electron micrographic study. *Blood, 28*:83–93, 1966.

136. Brooks, R. E. and Siegel, B. V.: Normal human lymph node cells: An electron microscopic study. *Blood, 27*:687–705, 1966.

137. Lennert, K, Caesar, R., and Müller, H. K.: Electron microscopic studies of germinal centers in man. In Cottier, H. *et al.: Germinal Centers in Immune Responses.* New York, Springer-Verlag, 1967, pp. 49–59.

138. Zucker-Franklin, D.: The ultrastructure of lymphocytes. *Sem Hemat, 6*:4–27, 1969.

Section 2

THE TROPHIC FUNCTION OF THE THYMUS
AND SMALL LYMPHOCYTES

Many researchers have suspected that the thymus holds the key to unlock many obscure compartments of the lymphocyte mystery. Therefore, having correlated evidence to indicate that the function of lymphoid elements is basically trophic, let us explore how this point of view stands in the light of recent experimental data. These data have accumulated very rapidly, owing to a general surge of interest in the thymus and the small lymphocytes, particularly as they relate to tissue transplantation and homograft rejection. The ensuing analysis will involve review of data which show that obliteration of the lymphoid tissue mass and the small lymphocytes by experimental methods, such as neonatal thymectomy, ionizing radiation, or immunosuppressive drugs, results in failure of growth in young animals or aberrations of growth in adults. By obliteration of the lymphoid elements, then, one may prove that their normal function is, indeed, trophic (as well as immunologic). Another aspect will be review of the data which indicate that small lymphocytes function as stem cells, along with the corresponding data that they function as donors of nucleoplasm rich in DNA. Through analysis of the quantitites involved, it will be shown why the popular stem cell hypothesis is quite unlikely. Also, the analysis will include an exposition of how the thymus gland and the small lymphocytes, as preeminent donors of nucleoplasm, not only feed other cells with valuable substrate but also feed them with information and energy essential to normal growth, normal resilience to stress and normal capacity to repair the damage produced by various forms of injury, such as trauma, infection, and grafting of genetically incompatible cells. Finally, there will ensue brief discussion on how the thymus gland may function as an endocrine organ.

Chapter 13

BACKGROUND MATERIAL

A T THE TIME of birth in higher orders of air-breathing vertebrates, particularly in humans, the thymus gland ranks next after the brain, liver, kidneys, and heart as being the largest single organ in the body.[1] Subsequently, it gradually shrinks in size relative to the total body mass and to the remaining lymphoid tissue mass but at the same time continues growth to attain greatest actual size at the time of puberty.[2-4] After the prepubertal period of rapid body growth has subsided, the gland gradually undergoes atrophy.[2-4] The gland differs from remaining definitive lymphoid organs of mammals in that it is derived from entoderm, as well as from mesenchyme.[2-5] Its entodermal cells are stranded from the vestigial respiratory epithelium of the embryonal gill system in a manner similar to the neighboring thyroid and parathyroid glands.[6] Differing from the latter, the thymic entodermal cells become so densely encased in lymphoid tissue that the gland is often called a lymphoepithelial organ.[2-7] Its lymphoid cells, like those of the gastrointestinal submucosa, are closely apposed to the entodermal cells [2-7] and lie in a position to be greatly affected by molecules excreted or secreted from them. The gland differs from other lymphoid organs not only in its entodermal cell population but also in that it contains a relatively dense population of small, cytoplasm-poor lymphocytes.[2-8] It is very significant [9,10] that, calculated in terms of DNA-bound phosphorus [11] (see Tables VI–VIII), the DNA concentration in thymic tissue is roughly 1½ times that in the nodes, 2 times that in the small bowel, 2 to 4 times that in the spleen and 5 to 50 times that in remaining tissues of the body. It is physiologically significant that during stress the thymus exceeds but shares with the remaining lymphoid tissues the propensity to involute or shrink rapidly.[12] It is clinically noteworthy that stress involution fails to occur in sudden, unexplained death [13] and that abnormally large thymus glands are prone to be associated with myasthenia gravis.[14] While the thymus has long been considered to have an ill-defined function somehow related to growth,[4] only recently has it been shown by experiments with thymic extracts [15-17] and by studies employing thymectomy followed by thymic reimplantation within millipore diffusion envelopes [18-21] that the thymic entoderm appears to produce a hormone which accelerates nucleic acid synthesis, growth, and immunologic function in lymphoid tissues and small lymphocytes. The mechanism whereby interaction between thymic entodermal cells and lymphoid cells becomes translated into accelerated lymphoid tissue growth, general body growth, and immunologic competence remains to be settled.

It seems clear that small lymphocytes, both within and outside the thymus are critically involved in such end functions. Therefore, the problem of thymic function may be approached in terms of small lymphocytes and their function. At present, predominant theories of thymic function are based on the popular but not universally accepted premise that small lymphocytes are

These tables are reproduced through the courtesy of Academic Press Inc. and the late I. Leslie (see Ref. 11).* Attention is directed particularly toward the columns encased in heavier lines. Here it will be noted that the tissue concentration of DNA-P varies in different tissues, the lymphoid tissues (especially the thymus) having relatively great concentrations. While the DNA-P content of mammalian cells is roughly equal (see 9th column of the tables), its concentration in cells or tissues is a direct reflection of cell size. Small cells, such as small lymphocytes with little cytoplasm, have relatively high concentrations of DNA-P. Tissues made up of small cells, such as small lymphocytes, have relatively high concentrations of DNA-P.

The RNA-P concentrations in different tissues varies (see 4th column), and depends not only on cell size, but also on intracytoplasmic concentration. Although the bulk of lymphoid cells possess relatively little cytoplasm, the lymphoid tissue concentration of RNA-P compares relatively well with remaining tissues, indicating a relatively high RNA-P concentration in many of the cells of which the lymphoid tissues are composed.

In Table VIII particular attention is directed also toward the loss of mass, RNA-P, and DNA-P in the spleen during protein deprivation (as compared with the loss in the liver and remaining tissues).

* The references included in the 10th columns of these tables are not included in this text, and can be found in Dr. Leslie's treatise.

TABLE VI
AMOUNTS OF RIBONUCLEIC ACID PHOSPHORUS (PNA-P) AND DEOXYRIBONUCLEIC ACID PHOSPHORUS (DNA-P) IN ADULT RAT TISSUES

Tissue	Weight of organ, g.	Total per organ		Micrograms per 100 mg. fresh tissue		Micrograms per mg. protein N		Picograms per average cell[b]		Ratio PNA-P/DNA-P	Refs.
		PNA-P	DNA-P	PNA-P	DNA-P	PNA-P	DNA-P	PNA-P	DNA-P		
Liver	7.67	7.19	1.66	93.4	21.6	36.9	8.6	4.0	0.913	4.38	(14)
				95	24					3.95	(1)
	12.0	9.21	2.02	77.5	16.8	33.5	7.25	5.25	1.14	4.62	(47)
	5.46	5.56	1.07	102	19.7	36.3	7.0			5.14	(48)
						34.8	10.6			3.28	(49)
Pancreas				198	48				0.712	4.1	(14, 37)
				178	45.2					3.96	(50)
Testis				41	23					1.78	(51)
Seminal vesicle		0.107	0.056	48.5	25.4					1.94	(52)
Small intestine				73.2	129.2				0.738	0.57	(14, 23)
Brain	1.52	0.56	0.21	36.8	13.8	25.4	9.2			2.67	48
				18.8	20.0					0.94	(37)
				13.5	9.4					1.43	(53)
				17.5	12.3					1.42	(50)
Lung				52.0	92.1				0.651	0.57	(14, 23)
				18.0	60.5					0.30	(50)
				36.0	71.0					0.5	(54)
Kidney[c]	0.73	0.480	0.195	65.7	26.7	27.3	11.3		0.652	2.46	(14, 48)
				40.7	41.8					0.97	(37)
				29.0	32.4					0.89	(55)
	0.694	0.484	0.213	69.7	30.7	34.3	15.1			2.27	(56)
Heart				31.4	30.6				0.627	1.03	(14, 57)
				12.4	14.5					0.85	(50)
Skeletal muscle[d]				6.7	5.7					1.17	(58)
				20	9.6					2.1	(53)
	7.41	1.80	0.37	24.5	5.0	38.6	7.9			4.9	(59)
Thymus				53	276				0.718	0.19	(14, 37)
				38	264					0.14	(50)
Spleen[e]				49.9	140				0.633	0.36	(14, 37)
	0.52	0.40	0.40	77	77	36.4	36.4			1.0	(60)
				86.4	84.1					1.03	(61)
				58	165					0.35	(54)
Bone marrow				87	153				0.670	0.57	(14, 51)
				126	130					0.97	(61)

TABLE VII
AMOUNTS OF RIBONUCLEIC ACID PHOSPHORUS (PNA-P) AND
DEOXYRIBONUCLEIC ACID PHOSPHORUS (DNA-P) IN VARIOUS
ANIMAL AND HUMAN TISSUES

Tissue and Species	Weight of organ, g.	Total per organ		Micrograms per 100 mg. fresh tissue		Micrograms per mg. protein N		Picograms per average cell		Ratio PNA-P/DNA-P	Refs.
		PNA-P	DNA-P	PNA-P	DNA-P	PNA-P	DNA-P	PNA-P	DNA-P		
Liver:											
Mouse				93.0	25.5	32.4	8.9			3.62	(62)
Mouse				92.9	27.9	28.1	8.4			3.34	(36)
Mouse				90.0	28.5					3.16	(63)
Mouse				92.7	23.2					4.00	(64)
Rabbit				79	17					4.6	(65)
Rabbit				30.9	7.3					4.26	(66)
Rabbit				31.9	16.1					1.98	(24)
Rabbit										1.41	(67)
Cat				78	34					2.30	(5)
Guinea pig				97	42					2.30	(53)
Pullets	45.0	37.8	14.0	84	31.1					2.70	(39)
Cockerel	37.8	29.3	15.6	77.5	41.3					1.86	(39)
Monkey				29	8.4					3.45	(68)
Man				52	21	21.4	8.8	2.48	1.0	2.48	(69)
Pancreas:											
Ox				100	6.5					15.4	(1)
Ox				177	22					8.1	(5)
Rabbit				119	52					2.3	(5)
Cat				146	43					4.3	(5)
Submaxillary gland:											
Mouse				88.0	58.3	62.5	41.5	2.01	1.34	1.51	(70)
Mouse	0.069	0.051	0.027	75.1	38.5					1.95	(71)
Kidney:											
Mouse										1.0	(62)
Mouse										1.16	(72)
Rabbit				16.7	12.5					1.34	(66)
Rabbit										0.54	(67)
Guinea pig				36	36					1.0	(53)
Man				20	16	27.2	21	1.10	0.83	1.33	(69)
Spleen:											
Mouse										0.30	(72)
Mouse										0.37	(62)
Rabbit										0.32	(67)
Guinea pig				71	91					0.8	(53)
Rabbit				73	91					0.8	(5)
Man				36	77					0.5	(5)

TABLE VII (*Continued*).

Tissue and Species	Weight of organ, g.	Total per organ PNA-P	Total per organ DNA-P	Micrograms per 100 mg. fresh tissue PNA-P	Micrograms per 100 mg. fresh tissue DNA-P	Micrograms per mg. protein N PNA-P	Micrograms per mg. protein N DNA-P	Picograms per average cell PNA-P	Picograms per average cell DNA-P	Ratio PNA-P/DNA-P	Refs.
Thymus:											
Mouse	0.033	0.020	0.086	62	262					0.24	(73)
Mouse										0.15	(72)
Calf				90	225					0.4	(5)
Lymphoid tissue:											
Mouse				52	180					0.29	(73)
Mouse										0.28	(72)
Bone marrow:											
Rabbit				18	48					0.38	(51)
Man				4.7	5.75			0.69	0.869	0.81	(74)
Leucocytes:											
Rabbit				22.5	95.1					0.24	(75)
Man								0.25	0.734	0.38	(74)
Brain:											
Rabbit										0.73	(67)
Dog, white matter				5.3	6.3					0.84	(76)
gray matter				11.1	5.3					2.10	(76)
Monkey, white matter				6.4	12.4					0.52	(77)
gray matter				11.5	9.6					1.20	(77)
Guinea pig				24	28					0.8	(53)
Sciatic nerve: Cat				3.9	4.8					0.9	(76)
Muscle:											
Rabbit				24	8					3.0	(65)
Rabbit										0.54	(67)
Guinea pig				24.5	10					2.45	(53)
Heart: Guinea pig				27	24					1.1	(53)
Skin: Mouse				11.9	39.3	7.6	25.0	0.22	0.71	0.30	(70)
Thyroid: pig										0.52	(78)
Crop gland: Pigeon	1.53	0.50	0.38	32.6	25.1					1.30	(79)
Brain:											
Carp						20.6	16.0	0.45	0.35	1.28	(80)
Tortoise						29.6	9.1	1.63	0.50	3.26	
Duck						10.6	6.3	0.44	0.26	1.69	
Fowl						17.0	8.3	0.45	0.22	2.05	
Rat						9.7	8.2	0.72	0.61	1.18	
Guinea pig						18.5	7.9	1.61	0.69	2.33	
Cat						8.9	7.8	0.79	0.69	1.14	
Dog						8.2	7.0	0.79	0.67	1.18	
Man						27.4	7.1	2.63	0.68	3.87	

conducive to the growth of lymphocytes, at least in the fishes, and possibly in all embryos as they pass through the gill stage within the aqueous environment of the egg. The primordial mesenchyme of the thymus, which is also developing in close relation to the gill arches (which are the first arterial vessels to develop in the embryo), will commence its differentiation under conditions of relatively high oxygen concentration and will continue to do so as the gills become vestigial and the thymic epithelium becomes stranded into the neck in close relation to the derivatives of the gill arches (which are all the arteries proximal to the ductus arteriosus and are arteries preferentially treated with respect to oxygenation during the evolution of complex shunting patterns which take place during embryogenesis).[6,150]

Third, the rate of development of the thymus far outstrips that of the remaining lymphoid organs, so that at the time of birth in mammals, it has attained the relatively great size and many other unique characeristics alluded to earlier. Such a rapid rate of development is undoubtly owing to its close functional relationship with the thymic epithelium. It remains to be determined, however, whether the thymic epithelium serves as a source of lymphoid stem cells, as argued by some (see Chap. 16, B), or as the source of a hormone which accelerates the growth of lymphocytes in a favorable tissue location with respect to oxygen tension—a theme which will be developed further.

It has long been known that in long-necked birds such as the chicken a lymphoid organ histologically similar to the thymus develops in an embryologically analogous manner by stranding of entodermal cells from a cloacal pouch, called the bursa of Fabricius.[7] Quite recently it has been found that extirpation of this lymphoid organ in the neonatal chick will result in an immunologic disorder which differs from neonatal thymectomy (in the same species) in that antibody production appears more profoundly impaired than does immunologic response involving the reaction of "immunologically competent" small lymphocytes.[24-26] Because of the therapeutic desirability of eliminating cellular immune responses but retaining humoral antibody responses in transplant recipients, the relationship between the bursa of

Fabricius and the thymus has been the subject of intensive study all over the world and especially by Dr. R. A. Good and his group at the University of Minnesota. Although a comparable lymphoid organ remains to be found in the rectal area of mammals, active search continues for a true counterpart higher in the gastrointestinal tract.[24-27]

Very recently it came to my attention and it was reported [47] (and see Letter to the Editor, *Blood, 33*:261, 1969) that in long-necked amphibians such as the turtle, the bursa of Fabricius functions as a gill, carrying on respiratory gas exchange when the turtle sucks water in and out of the cloaca. It allows the turtle to remain submerged for relatively long periods of time. Although all vertebrates develop in the aquatic environment of the egg or of the fetal sac inside the womb, it is not clear to what extent the gill pouches function as gills during development, especially in placentates.*

However, if one looks upon the bursa of Fabricius as a gill equivalent, one may look upon the entodermal cells stranded from there as equivalent to the entodermal cells stranded from the gill pouches in the neck. As the latter, after becoming stranded, continue onward to become the endocrine cells of the thymus, thyroid, and parathyroid glands, one may suspect that the entodermal cells stranded from the cloacal bursa assume an endocrine function equivalent to the entodermal cells of one or more of these glands. Moreover, because these particular glands are similarly derived from an organ formerly concerned with

---

* It seems clear that whether within the egg shell or in the womb, all developing embryos must breathe. Moreover, throughout embryonal life in oviparous species and prior to placentation in mammals, the embryos must breathe in a liquid medium where respiration via gills may prove advantageous and efficient. Of course, in mammals wherein nidation and placentation occur relatively early in the span of embryonal life, neither branchial nor cloacal gills would seem necessary for a prolonged period, owing to the fact that respiration (oxygenation) is established relatively early via the placenta. It is perhaps for this reason that the middle branchial pouches have received attention primarily as sources of endocrine epithelium in the lower neck, rather than as respiratory epithelia. For similar reasons, perhaps, a cloacal bursa concerned either with respiration or with endocrine differentiation remains to be identified in mammals.

In oviparous species, however, respiration must continue via the vitelline membranes, via the branchial gills, via cloacal gills, or through all, while the growing embryo "swims" suspended in the egg. In those oviparous species whose eggs hatch under water, the branchial gills continue as the principal organ of respiration, as in fishes and frogs (before metamorphosis). Such species, among other attributes, have relatively short necks and hearts whose outflow tracts are relatively close to the branchial gills. In those oviparous species whose eggs hatch in air, the branchial gills give way to the lungs and the endocrine organs of the lower neck by the time of hatching, as in snakes, turtles, birds, and monotremes. Out of the latter, the turtles and birds (such as chickens) are of particular interest, having in common relatively long necks and hearts whose outflow tracts become elongated from the branchial gills with growth of the neck. In these species, one finds a well-developed cloacal bursa which continues to function as an auxiliary respiratory organ (in the turtle), or as an auxiliary endocrine organ quite similar to the thymus (in birds). One wonders, therefore, if the relative importance of the cloacal bursa as an auxiliary gill or as an auxiliary thymus-like gland may not be a function of the relative distance the heart has to pump blood to be aerated at external openings of the embryonal body during that period of embryogenesis when the neck is elongating and the lungs are developing but not yet functional.

respiration, it would seem reasonable to suspect that when the submerged, gill-breathing vertebrate with a soft, cartilaginous skeleton undergoes metamorphosis into a land-roving, air-breathing one with a hard, calcified skeleton that their endocine function will continue closely related. Noting that the endocrine cells of thymus, thyroid, and parathyroids appear to have something to do with DNA synthesis, oxygen utilization, and calcium-phosphorous utilization, respectively, and that they all appear to enhance lymphocytopoiesis in the thymus,[2-4] one may suspect that all are concerned with oxidative chain phosphorylations leading to DNA synthesis in lymphocytes.

With such conventional as well as obtuse background material in mind, let us proceed to explore how the thymus and the small lymphocytes are interrelated and do so with particular emphasis on Lavoisier's principles of mass and energy conservation.

Chapter 14

THE SPECIFIC METHOD OF APPROACH

S INCE IT REMAINS to be settled whether small lymphocytes function as stem cells or as trephocytes and it remains to be settled whether the thymus produces a hormone which merely accelerates lymphocyte growth or whether it confers immunologic capacity on small lymphocytes by some other mechanism, the specific method of approach will be via the logical method of starting with a premise, testing whether the premise will explain the observed effects of thymectomy, analyzing arguments against and counterarguments for the premise, and then reducing competing arguments to the point of absurdity. The premise is as follows: *Normally the thymic entodermal cells produce a hormone which enhances nucleic acid synthesis in lymphoid tissues locally and generally, whereas the latter respond by accelerating the production of small lymphocytes which donate nucleic acids to other cells.*

free living controls, their lymphoid tissue mass and circulating small lymphocyte mass are smaller, and their growth rate correspondingly slower. Perhaps the lack of wasting or "runt disease" in neonatally thymectomized axenic animals is owing to the fact that such animals are effectively isolated from organisms (pathogenic and saprophytic) which compete for substrate and would ordinarily produce rapid wasting and death in neonatally thymectomized, immunologically deficient, free-living animals.

Favoring the trophic concept vs. the stem cell hypothesis is that whether or not immunologic competence is attained, the lymphoid tissue mass and circulating small lymphocyte mass are only smaller, not absent, in axenic animals.[65-68] Sufficient small lymphocytes are already present in the body prior to and subsequent to neonatal thymectomy to theoretically increase the lymphocyte population ad infinitum, provided the small lymphocytes actually function as stem cells. Therefore, it must be and has been postulated [16,18-21,23-27] that the thymus not only supplies a critical stem cell mass to colonize other lymphoid tissues but also a factor essential to the maturation of such stem cells (or similar stem cells from other sources) [27] into immunologically competent cells. Although all agree that this factor emanates from the thymic entodermal cells, it is not settled how the factor operates (cf. Refs. 16–21, 23–27) and why the factor is no longer necessary after a critical peripheral lymphoid tissue mass is attained during neonatal life and as long as this mass remains intact during adult life (cf. Chap. 15).

Thus, results obtained from the study of neonatally thymectomized, axenic animals do not really clarify whether the thymocytes actually colonize other lymphoid tissues or whether they donate substances such as DNA, essential to their growth and function. The fact that neonatal removal of the thymus gland (before a critical peripheral lymphoid tissue mass is attained) results in slowed neonatal growth rate can be interpreted to indicate that the function of the thymus as a whole is trophic, not only toward remaining lymphoid tissues but also toward the body as a whole.

B. STUDIES ON CHROMOSOME MARKERS *IN VIVO*

Following the infusion of donor thoracic duct lymphocytes or implantation of donor thymus into a host having a chromosomal karyotype different from the donor, the blood and lymphoid tissues of an irradiated (or syngeneic, immunologically tolerant) host are found to become populated by lymphocytes possessing the distinctive donor karyotype (e.g. Y chromosome).[69,70] Moreover, following the infusion of minced myeloid tissue or spleen from a donor into a sublethally irradiated host, the bone marrow and lymphoid organs become populated by myeloid and lymphoid cells with chromosomal karyotype distinctive of the donor.[71] Separately and together, such experimental observations lend strong support to the stem cell hypothesis, the current interpretation being that hemopoietic stem cells (presumably small lymphocytes) from the donor recirculate, colonize, replicate, and differentiate within the host, thus supplying an obvious need for new blood cells of various types.[23,72]

Related experimental observations may controvert this interpretation and simultaneously support the trophic concept of DNA donation. Even when there is no obvious need for new blood cells of various types, as in an unirradiated human, there follows the infusion of lymphocytes of foreign, distinctive karyotype an unexplained lag period of some 12 hours, during which no lymphocytes of foreign karyotype can be identified in the peripheral blood.[73] This lag is not particularly consistent with the lymphocyte recirculation theory. After 12 hours, and persisting up to 10 days, three to seven times as many lymphocytes of foreign karyotype are found in the vascular system as can be accounted for by the number of lymphocytes in the inoculum. The number within the organized lymphoid tissues, which normally contain on the order of 100 times as many lymphocytes as the vascular system,[74] is unknown. After 10 days, all the lymphocytes of foreign karyotype disappear[73] (without overt systemic reaction). Such findings are theoretically explained[72-73] on the basis that the infused foreign lymphocytes are initally trapped in lymphoid organs, such as the spleen, and there undergo dedifferentiation, replication, and after the lag period (which seems relatively short with strated conclusively,[23,83] because it is not clear whether the pyroninophilic cells appearing within the organized lymphoid tissues after any form of antigenic stimulation (including PHA) are differentiated from small migratory lymphocytes, from fixed cells in the reticular stroma or from the integrated activity of both.

2. *In vivo* PHA injections thus far have failed to elicit any consistent, clinically beneficial specific immunologic or hemopoietic response.

3. In tissue culture systems, PHA-stimulated lymphocytes not only fail to differentiate into anything other than plasmacyte-like cells and atypical macrophages [23,84] but also fail to produce specific antibodies to a new antigen without addition of previously sensitized macrophages to the culture system.[61]

4. Electron micrographic studies on PHA-stimulated lymphocytes shed some doubt on the transformation of relatively large numbers of inoculated small lymphocytes and thus far seem in keeping with adaptation to culture conditions of small numbers of cells which replicate at rates sufficient to explain the numbers of cells appearing to be transformed.[84] In the body, disappearance of marrow lymphocytes signals the erythropoietic response to anoxia.[85]

5. Although some lymphocytes undergo morphologic transformation in tissue culture systems, many of the inoculated lymphocytes disintegrate.[23,82,84,86] The numbers being transformed appear roughly proportional to the numbers which disintegrate, with few undergoing transformation when few disintegrate.[86] If nucleic acids from the latter are reutilized by the former, their impact on the rate and form of growth must be taken into account. It was shown by Carrel [40] many years ago that one of the best ways to make mammalian cells grow in tissue culture is to add leukocytes (lymphocytes).

6. Observations that lymphocyte transformation is accelerated also by antigens to which the donor has been sensitized previously [23,87] indicate that the small lymphocytes are not necessarily undifferentiated stem cells but cells, many of which during their formative stages in the lymphoid organs of the body are provided

with very specific informational codes in their DNA.

7. Observations that small lymphocytes stimulated by PHA or antigens in tissue culture systems resume DNA, RNA, and cytoplasmic protein synthesis do not necessarily indicate that small lymphocytes are stem cells for plasmacytes or any other specific type of blood cell for at least three reasons. First, lymphocytes in tissue culture fail to develop into other types of cells resembling granulocytes, erythrocytes, or megakaryocytes.[23] Second, lymphocytes themselves normally pass through a pyroninophilic stage during the course of their normal development *in vivo*. Therefore, should they all be called plasmacytes during this stage? If the von Marschalkó plasmacyte is considered to be typical of the mature stage of plasmacytic development and the stage where one identifies pyroninophilic precursors as being plasmacytes, relatively few transformed lymphocytes would be identified as definitive plasmacytes in tissue culture systems. (The argument here, of course, revolves about how a plasmacyte is to be morphologically defined, after von Marschalkó, or after Unna? (see Sect. 1).) Third, it can be argued whether the resumption of DNA, RNA, new cytoplasmic protein synthesis, and mitosis is a true indication of "dedifferentiation," or whether it is owing to derepression of certain chromosomal characteristics of living cells (cf. Frenster[88]) in tissue culture systems.*

8. Careful scrutiny of photomicrographs showing lymphocytes stimulated in tissue culture systems will reveal that the transformed cells demonstrate relatively prolific cytoplasmic shedding. Therefore, it should be questioned whether such cells are merely producing antibodies or whether they are attempting to produce plasma (see Sects. 1 and 3).

9. The morphologic appearance of lymphocytes stimulated by the mitogen PHA is similar to that observed in malignant lymphoma cells and reminiscent of that reported in tissue culture of

---

* In other words, are the small peripheral blood lymphocytes in PHA culture systems really undergoing differentiation into stem cells for plasmacytes? Or, as a result of de-repression of certain nuclear enzymes, are they merely resuming functional attributes present during earlier stages of their own development in organized lymphoid tissues, i.e. reutilization of DNA from other cells, DNA synthesis, mitosis, RNA synthesis, cytoplasmic protein production, production of relatively specific agglutinins, cytoplasmic shedding, plasma production, etc?

other types of seemingly differentiated cells rendered malignant-appearing after incorporation of P_v or SV-40 viral DNA.[89] Thus it should be questioned whether the lymphocytes are being stimulated into a purposeful or into a malignant transformation in which respiration is carried on by anaerobic glycolysis.*

10. Recently it has been shown that lymphocyte transformation in tissue culture can be induced by heterologous lymphocytes † and by disrupted heterologous lymphocytes.[23] Even more recently, it has been shown that lymphocyte transformation in tissue culture can be induced by E-B viruses and that after incorporation of the viral DNA, many of the lymphocytes in mitosis have altered or abnormal chromosomes.[90] The latter observation suggests that in cultured human lymphocytes, as in cultures of bacteria and other kinds of mammalian cells, heterologous DNA can be incorporated into the chromosomes and that its incorporation may result in altered chromosomal characteristics, as well as altered growth characteristics.

Such *in vitro* observations lend support to the consideration in the previous section on chromosomal markers that DNA from some lymphocytes may become incorporated into the DNA of other proliferating lymphocytes and that the expression of its code may result in altered chromosomal characteristics in the latter. Whereas the *in vitro* studies indicate that such genetic hybridization can occur, the *in vivo* studies on chromosome markers may be interpreted to indicate that it occurs in quantity before the heterologous DNA is recognized as foreign and rejected or when the subject is immunologically paralyzed.

11. Many years after irradiation of various segments of the body, the peripheral blood lymphocytes subjected to PHA stimulation in tissue culture systems may show chromosomal aberrations induced by the irradiation.[279] This finding has led many to conclude that some of the peripheral blood lymphocytes are of

---

* For preliminary data on lactic acid production and the effect of carbon dioxide tension on the relative rates of lymphocyte transformation vs. disintegration in PHA systems, cf. Wilson and Thompson.[86]

† The quantitative induction of lymphocyte transformation by heterologous lymphocytes in tissue culture currently serves as the basis for one form of histocompatibility testing prior to organ transplantation.[23]

very prolonged biologic life and that they may recirculate almost indefinitely,[280] an interpretation compatible with the stem cell hypothesis. However, analysis of the rate at which lymphcytes with abnormal chromosomes make their appearance in the peripheral blood following repeated doses of irradiation will reveal that a plateau is reached at about 10 days [281] (i.e. about the same time that the primary immunologic response comes to full fruition) (see Chap. 18). If the number of lymphocytes in peripheral blood with abnormal chromosomes is dose related and their biologic life prolonged, one should expect their number to rise in linear fashion. The plateau at 10 days, then, may be interpreted to indicate that many are of relatively short biologic life and that the DNA from some is selectively reutilized and expressed for prolonged periods of time in subsequent generations of lymphocytes.

1. Summary

Thus the study of lymphocyte transformation in tissue culture has led to an important series of observations whose application to what actually happens *in vivo* is open to various interpretations. This form of study is unique in comparison with the study of lymphocytes in the living subject because the cultured cells are not subject to the controls normally imposed by interaction with other types of cells, especially stromal cells of mesenchymal derivation, and the controls imposed by substances contantly being supplied and being taken away by the circulating plasma. As in the heavily irradiated or neonatally thymectomized animal, they grow in an environment where the continual addition of endogenous lymphocytes from various lymphoid organs is effectively eliminated and in an environment in which they are on their own insofar as their immunologic role is concerned.

Viewed under such conditions, the stem cell hypothesis of small lymphocyte function is favored by the facts that some lymphocytes demonstrate resumption of nucleic acid synthesis; that many of the latter morphologically resemble blast cells, and that they may synthesize agglutinins directed toward antigens to which the donor has been sensitized previously. The trophic concept is favored by the facts that some of the lymphocytes disintegrate, that irregardless of previous sensitization, some of the transforming cells appear to shed cytoplasm which may be interpreted to indicate resumption of plasma secretion (see Sect. 1), and that disintegration and shedding is associated with an increased rate of transformation and growth in some of the lymphocytes in the culture medium.

If one chooses the latter interpretation, the consequences of lymphocyte donation of DNA to other lymphocytes and the changes which may be wrought in the latter when this DNA is incorporated are of fundamental biological significance.

D. MICROBIOLOGIC STUDIES ON THYMIC AND BURSAL DEVELOPMENT

The following experimental results, particularly as interpreted by Dr. R. A. Good et al.,[24-26] have profoundly affected current concepts of lymphocytes as they relate to hemopoiesis as well as to immunity. First, it was found by Auerbach [91] that thymic entodermal explants microsurgically removed from the fetal mouse after 12 days' gestation are capable of differentiating into lymphocytes when transplanted into mouse anterior eye chambers, onto chick chorioallantoic membranes, and onto tissue culture media. Such explants were considered to be devoid of lymphocytes and consisted of stranded entodermal cells encased in a thin layer of mesenchyme. When the latter was eliminated by tryptic digestion and the explants were transplanted onto tissue culture media in which mesenchyme from other sources was present but separated from the entodermal transplants by millipore diffusion filters, it was found that adjacent mesenchyme was essential to normal entodermal differentiation and that the differentiation of lymphocytes proceeded from the transplanted entodermal cells. Second, it was shown by Ruth et al.[92] that the normal rate of lymphocyte development in the lymphoepithelial organs (including the thymus of mammals and the bursa of Fabricius of chickens), the normal rate of development of other lymphoid organs, and the development of immunologic reactivity in the small mammals and chickens is dependent on an interaction between the epithelial and the mesenchymal derivatives in such lymphoepithelial organs. Third, it was found by Ackerman and Knouff [93] that the development of lymphocytes in relation to the bursa of Fabricius of developing chickens is entirely analogous to that which takes place in relation to the thymus of developing mammals. Their electron microscopic studies and special staining techniques indicated entodermal derivation of the lymphocytes. Finally, it was noted that bursectomy in the neonatal chick results in a syndrome characterized by deficient humoral antibody production, whereas neonatal thymectomy in the same species results in a syndrome characterized predominantly by delayed cutaneous sensitivity reactions and delayed graft rejection.[24-26]

It was interpreted, therefore, that the entodermal derivation of the lymphocytes in these lymphoepithelial organs is indicative of special function, and proposed that the thymic lymphocytes appear specifically concerned with (small-lymphocyte–mediated) cellular immunity, whereas bursal lymphocytes (or bursa-like equivalents in mammals) appear specifically concerned with (plasmacyte-mediated) humoral immunity.[24-26] Moreover, because it was found that infusion of isotope-labeled thymus lymphocytes results in characteristic labeling of lymphocytes in other lymphoid, especially the spleen and liver,[94] it was proposed [24] and it remains a popular concept that the thymic and bursal lymphocytes function as stem cells which peripheralize (migrate from their site of origin) to circulate, colonize, and produce small immunologically competent lymphocytes and plasmacytes, respectively, in the other lymphoid tissues. Such interpretations of these data not only reinforce the stem cell concept of small lymphocyte function but also imply specialization of certain lymphocytes to specific immunologic functions. As an almost casual review of the current literature will attest, such interpretations have stimulated much related experimental research, many modified concepts, and a host of new terms to describe the functional roles of lymphocytes of various size and morphologic description.

The following considerations are against such a specific stem cell concept.

1. The entodermal derivation of thymic lymphocytes has long

been,[2-7,16] and remains,[91-97] a subject of dispute. Those continuing to advocate the common mesenchymal derivation of thymic lymphocytes and lymphocytes in other lymphoid organs of mammals point out that thymic explants in the mouse fetus of 12 days' gestation already contain lymphocyte precursor cells of mesenchymal derivation at the time of explantation [97] and that the relatively rapid rate of lymphocytopoiesis in close physical relation to such entodermal cells, both *in vivo* and *in vitro,* can be explained by the entodermal production of a hormone which accelerates lymphocytopiesis [96] (e.g. the lymphocytosis-stimulating factor (L.S.F.) of Metcalf [15] or the lymphotrophic hormone described by Goldstein *et al.*[17]).

2. A true counterpart of the bursa of Fabricius remains to be demonstrated in mammals, particularly if one considers the bursa to be a gill equivalent.[47] Therefore, it seems premature to designate some of the lymphocytes of mammals as being derived from the bursa, being derived from a bursa-like organ, or being bursa dependent, even though there is ample evidence to indicate that the mononuclear cell populations in the medullary reticulum of the nodes and spleen appear to react to antigenic stimuli earlier and in a fashion different from the mononuclear cell populations of the lymph follicles in these organs (see below, E, and Chap. 18, B).

3. As mentioned by Fichtelius and Bryant,[94] it is not certain whether the isotope labeling observed in lymphocytes of extra-thymic lymphoid organs is owing to peripheralization, circulation, colonization, and proliferation of infused, labeled, intact small thymic lymphocytes or owing to their donation of labeled DNA which becomes reutilized and incorporated within proliferating lymphocytes in other lymphoid organs, as well as in other rapidly growing cells such as fibroblasts, regenerating liver cells, and small intestinal epithelium. Metcalf [16] maintains and has presented evidence to prove that few, if any, small thymic lymphocytes leave the gland as intact cells under experimental conditions.

Moreover, if small thymic lymphocytes actually peripheralize, circulate, colonize, and proliferate, one should expect infusion of thymic, thoracic duct, or blood lymphocytes to effectively repopulate other lymphoid organs under experimental conditions and to do so with cells which can be recognized by labels other than isotopes, such as genotypic labels. Not only do infusions of thymic, thoracic duct, or peripheral blood lymphocytes of foreign karyotype fail to produce effective repopulation of the lymphoid organs and bone marrow of sublethally irradiated animals, but also prove much less effective than infusions of minced bone marrow or spleen in repopulating the thymus, bone marrow, and other lymphoid organs with cells of foreign karyotype under the same experimental conditions.[23,27]

The relative importance of stromal elements in such infusions is perhaps best emphasized in Downey's studies which not only showed the mesenchymal derivation of lymphocytes in many kinds of lymphoid organs but also presented evidence to prove that regenerating small lymphocytes in the thymus of irradiated mammals (including humans) are derived from mesenchymal reticular cells rather than from epithelial reticular cells.[95]

4. Finally, the stem cell and immunologic specificity of morphologically indistinct groups of small lymphocytes should be questioned if one places importance on their common mesenchymal derivation, their identical morphologic appearance, and their universal disintegration during stress—a condition wherein such specific stem cell and immunologic functions both would seem effectively obliterated by their disintegration.

Thus, the recent experimental findings on thymic development in relation to lymphocytopoiesis can be interpreted either in favor of the stem cell hypothesis or in favor of the trophic concept, depending on the position one takes with respect to the evidence for (a) the entodermal derivation of thymic lymphocytes vs. the entodermal production of a hormone which accelerates lymphocytopoiesis and (b) the concept of peripheralization, circulation, colonization, and proliferation of small lymphocytes from the thymus and other lymphoid organs vs. the donation of DNA by such cells to be reutilized in other proliferating lymphoid and nonlymphoid cells.

E. THE TRACING OF DNA PRECURSOR UTILIZATION WITH ISOTOPES

Observations that compounds containing radioactive isotopes are utilized in cells like chemically identical compounds made up of naturally occurring, relatively stable elements have been invaluable to the study of cellular growth and differentiation *in vivo*. Thus, when DNA precursor compounds such as phosphate containing radioactive phosphorous ($^{32}PO_4$) or thymidine containing tritium (^3HT) are introduced, they become incorporated into the DNA of growing cells, proportional to their concentration relative to the available concentration of identical naturally occurring, nonradioactive radicals or compounds. By measuring the quantity of isotope-labeled precursor incorporated into nuclei per unit of time, usually by scintillator counting of ionizations or by autoradiography (recording ionizations on X-ray film), the rate of DNA synthesis, and hence the rate of cell growth, can be estimated,[98-107] provided the concentrations of isotope-labeled precursors and unlabeled, naturally occurring precursors are constant relative to one another. By plotting the percentages of cells labeled up to and beyond peak labeling, the life span of given cell populations can be estimated,[98-107] provided the rate of cell birth and cell death remain in equilibrium throughout the period of study.

Interpretations of the cell growth or "kinetic" data obtained by isotope-labeling techniques are based on the following assumptions: [103,106-107]

1. The isotope-labeled precursor compound, particularly tritiated thymidine (^3HT), is nonexchangeable after the nuclear DNA is labeled.

2. DNA turnover is owing solely to cell division or to cell death.

3. Cellular reutilization of the labeled substance, particularly ^3HT, is negligible.

4. DNA synthesis indicates imminent cell division.

5. Ionizations from the relatively small quantity of isotope incorporated from such radicals or compounds does not damage the cells.

6. After intravenous injection, labeled nucleic acid precursors such as $^{32}PO_4$ and ^3HT, being relatively small molecules in comparison with proteins, are uniformly dispersed throughout the intravascular, interstitial, and intracellular fluids within a relatively short period of time. Since all body cells have equal opportunity to utilize these labeled (injected) precursors along with identical, unlabeled (endogenous) precursors, the rate and intensity of labeling will directly reflect the rate of DNA synthesis and growth over a period of time in a given cell population and the relative rates of DNA synthesis and growth in different cell populations of the body at any given time.

While all such assmputions are in jeopardy, assumptions 3 and 6 will be particularly singled out for challenge here.

1. Methods of Study, Findings, and Current Interpretations

When $^{32}PO_4$ or ^3HT is introduced intravenously in a single (or "flash") injection, different kinds of body cells incorporate the labeled precursor in their nuclei at various rates. The nuclei which incorporate the isotope most rapidly are those of the entodermal cells of the crypts of Lieberkuhn in the small intestine,[108-110] the precursor cells of granulocytes and erythrocytes in the bone marrow,[111-112] and the large and medium-sized lymphocytes of the thymus, spleen, bone marrow, lymph nodes, and Peyers patches of the small intestine.[98-110] The nuclei of such cells commence to incorporate the labeled radicals or compounds within minutes or hours, whereas the nuclei of cells comprising the mucosal and epithelial surfaces show evidence of isotope incorporation in hours or days.[98-112] Some cells, such as hepatic polygonal cells, brain cells, and muscle cells show very little evidence of isotope incorporation in their nuclei and are calculated, therefore, to be of prolonged biologic life with a slow or negligible rate of cell turnover.[108-110] Most of the early nuclear labeling after the injection of $^{32}PO_4$ or ^3HT takes place in the cells of lymphoid organs and, as evaluated by ^3HT grain counting, more or less in the following decremental order per quantity of tissue: thymus, lymphoid tissue of the bone marrow, spleen, peripheral lymph nodes, mesenteric nodes, and submucosal lymphoid tissue of the intestine.[98,112,113]

Prior to the accumulation of such data on lymphoid cells relative to other body cells, it was found by labeling with $^{32}PO_4$ and ^{14}C-labeled amino acids that the lymphoid organs in general and the lymphocytes specifically were soaking up inordinate quantities of isotope-labeled cell protein precursors (as measured by scintillation counting of cell suspensions or scintillation counting over selected body organs).[108-111] Radioactive phosphate proved to be a better label for studying lymphocytes than ^{14}C-labeled amino acids because of its relatively great concentration in nuclear DNA. But, owing to the fact that $^{32}PO_4$ is also incorporated into RNA and cytoplasmic proteins in lesser concentrations, ^{3}HT proved to be a more ideal DNA precursor for experimental study for the following reasons. First, it has a relatively great concentration in DNA, as opposed to its concentration in RNA, cytoplasmic proteins, and in the plasma. Also, being concentrated primarily in nuclei, its presence there could be detected by placing photographic emulsions over cell suspensions or tissue sections and recording with precision in which cells ionizations take place and how many ionizations are taking place per unit of time in different types of cells.

Radioactive phosphate, however, has theoretical advantages over tritiated thymidine, in that it is a smaller molecule* which may diffuse more rapidly. In addition, although it is less specific for nuclei than ^{3}HT and does not readily distinguish between the ionizations produced from nuclei of closely related cells, it does give a more direct and quantitative measurement of the total amount of precursor incorporated into cells of a given class chosen and studied by other methods, e.g. direct measurements of incorporation into measured weights or volumes of cells and tissues and direct measurements of $^{32}PO_4$ incorporated into DNA (DNA-P) fractions extracted from given tissues or cell concentrates.[113-115] Moreover, a great deal of the $^{32}PO_4$ data has been obtained from humans and large animals, whereas the ^{3}HT data

---

* $^{32}PO_4$ has a molecular weight of 96, whereas ^{3}HT has a molecular weight of 242.

has been obtained almost exclusively from experimental animals (the most accurate quantitative data having been obtained from rats). Therefore, both the $^{32}PO_4$ and ^3HT data will be considered here.

When $^{32}PO_4$ is infused intravenously into humans or into dogs, the lymphocytes obtained from the thoracic duct lymph and from peripheral blood start labeling within minutes and continue to label at linear rates which peak in the thoracic duct lymphocyte suspensions in 24 to 30 hours; and in peripheral blood lymphocyte concentrates at 2 to 4 days (see Figs. 35–36). Subsequently, the numbers of labeled lymphocytes fall off in the thoracic duct more rapidly than they do in the peripheral blood (an observation considered by Perry to mitigate against recirculation of lymphocytes from blood to thoracic duct lymph).[104] In the circulating blood, after a linear increase to a 2 to 4 day peak, the numbers of ^{32}P-labeled lymphocytes fall off relatively rapidly at first and continue to fall off in a declining exponential curve which plots to infinity, small numbers of labeled cells persisting for periods as long as 90 to 300 days.[116] By extrapolation, some of the curves are assumed to cross the baseline at 100 days in humans, thus giving an estimate of 100 days for the lifespan of some of the lymphocytes in the blood.[116]

Following single injections of ^3HT into rats, with simultaneous sampling of thoracic duct lymph and circulating blood, very similar curves were obtained [98,102,105-107,117] (see Figs. 37 and 38) but were obtained over a more extended period of time (perhaps owing to a slow rate of diffusion of ^3HT). Peak labeling of small lymphocytes in the thoracic duct occurred at 12 days, whereas peak labeling of the lymphocytes in the peripheral blood occurred somewhat later.[98,117] The labeling rate of lymphocytes in the peripheral blood was found to be faster than that in the thoracic duct lymph [98] (another observation mitigating against massive recirculation). In addition, it was noted that at about four to five days after the injection of ^3HT label, the straight linear rate of increase in labeled small lymphocytes began to deviate decrementally from the straight line in proportion to daily increase in body weight of the rats studied [98,117] (an observation

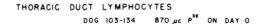

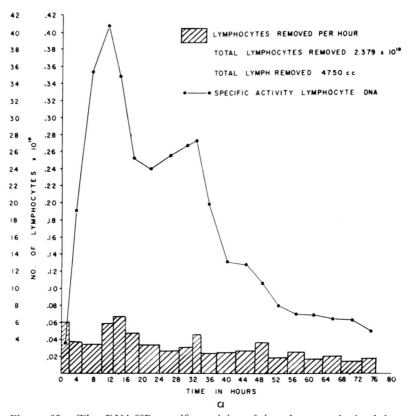

Figure 35*a*. The DNA-^{32}P specific activity of lymphocytes obtained by cannulation of the thoracic duct in dogs after intravenous injection of radioactive phosphate (^{32}PO$_4$). Note the linear rise to peak labeling at 8 to 12 hours and the declining exponential fall in labeling to low but significant levels. From Perry *et al*.[104]

which would lead one to suspect dilution of labeled precursors because if their concentration with respect to unlabeled precursors remained constant, their relative rates of utilization should remain the same).

By sampling the thymus gland simultaneously, it was found that the rate of increase in labeled small lymphocytes in the thymus

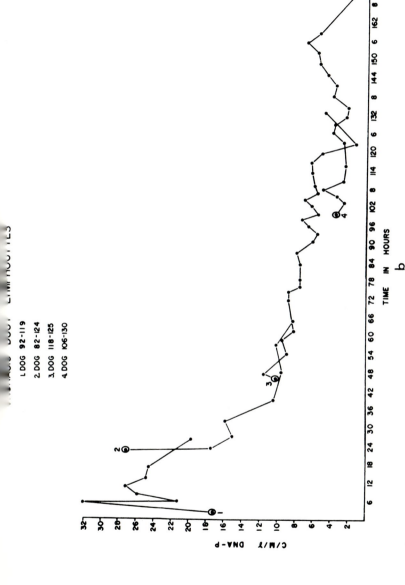

Figure 35*b*. The DNA-³²P specific activity of lymphocytes obtained by cannulation of the thoracic ducts in series of dogs with sampling at progressively longer intervals after the intravenous injection of ³²PO₄. Note again the declining exponential fall in relative number of lymphocytes labeled. From: Perry *et al.*[104]

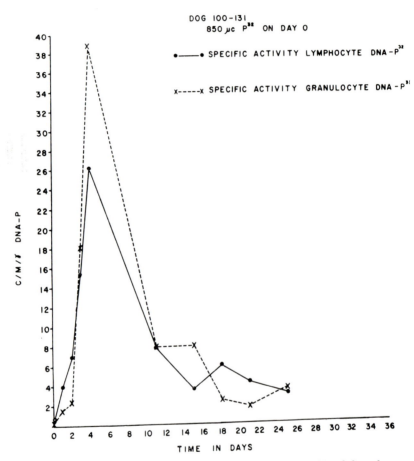

Figure 36. The DNA-^{32}P specific activity in peripheral blood lymphocytes and granulocytes in dogs after intravenous injection of [32]PO$_4$. Note again the linear rise to peak labeling and the declining exponential fall in labeled cells, possibly indicative of reutilization of the label. Note also the later time of peak labeling in lymphocytes from peripheral blood (4 days), as compared with thoracic duct lymph (see Figs. 35a and b From Perry et al.[104]

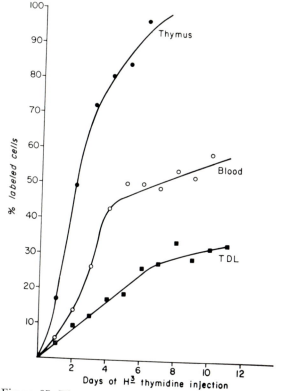

Figure 37. The rate of appearance of labeled small lymphocytes in the thymus, blood, and thoracic duct lymph (TDL) of rats after intramuscular injection of tritiated thymidine (^{3}HT). Although the time of peak labeling is not shown, note the gradual decline from a linear rate of labeling after four days. From Everett *et al.*[117]

far exceeds the rate of increase in labeling of similar cells in the thoracic duct lymph or circulating blood [98] (an observation suggesting to some that a large proportion of the lymphocytes in the peripheral blood and thoracic duct lymph originate in the thymus).

Finally, in these studies reported by Everett *et al.*,[98,117] it was found that the large and medium-sized lymphocytes in all the areas mentioned labeled earlier than the small lymphocytes.

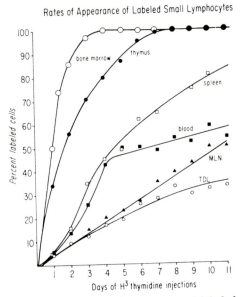

Figure 38. The rates of appearance of labeled small lymphocytes in the bone marrow, thymus, spleen, peripheral blood, mesenteric lymph nodes (MLN), and thoracic duct lymph (TDL) in rats after daily intramuscular injections of [3]HT. Although peak labeling and plateaus are reached in the bone marrow and thymus after four days, note the relatively slow rate of labeling in mesenteric nodes and thoracic duct lymph. From Everett and Tyler.[98]

(Labeled small lymphocytes were primarily counted.) Presuming that it takes a period of time for such cells to differentiate from their precursors, a part of the discrepancy in time between peak labeling with [32]PO$_4$ and [3]HT might be explained also on such grounds. The fall off a linear rate of labeling, as a function of time, made the time of peak labeling difficult to estimate after a single injection of [3]HT, particularly when different slopes were obtained from the different areas sampled (see Figs. 37 and 38).

As in the [32]PO$_4$ studies, it was found after single injections of [3]HT that the numbers of labeled lymphocytes in the circulating blood fall off at declining exponential rates, with small numbers of labeled cells persisting for prolonged periods of time.[105-107] Although distinct second appearance—disappearance curves of labeled cells were not constantly observed after single injections of $^{32}PO_4$[100,116] or ^{3}HT,[105-107] it was interpreted from such data that the blood contains two populations of small lymphocytes, one of rapid growth and short biologic life (e.g. 2–4 days)[100,105-107] and another with slower rate of growth and a prolonged but indefinite biologic life (e.g. 14–220 days).[98-103,105-107,111,117]

Such interpretations were challenged by Trowell[118] and Hamilton,[119] who maintained that the declining exponential rate of labeled lymphocyte disappearance in the circulating blood could be explained on the basis of reutilization of labeled precursors in the formation of additional new lymphocytes. Negating the latter interpretation of the isotope data and obviating the consideration of the time it takes for uniform dispersion of labeled precursor to take place in the body (cf. assumption 6), the techniques of spaced injections and continuous infusions of smaller quantities of ^{3}HT were employed by Everett *et al.*,[98,117] Little *et al.*,[106] and Robinson *et al.*[107] The emphasis in these studies was placed not upon the appearance—disappearance curves of labeled cells but upon how long it takes for unlabeled cells to disappear from different organs sampled and from the circulating blood. Everett *et al.* found that the rate of disappearance of unlabeled cells in the thymus was strictly linear (see Fig. 39), suggesting a random departure of unlabeled cells from the thymus[117] (to destinations unknown but possibly very significant). The significance of this observation will be considered later in a different context (cf. page 156).

Proof for existence of long-lived lymphocytes was presented by Little *et al.*,[106] and Robinson *et al.*,[107] who showed that with continuous infusions of ^{3}HT, unlabeled and poorly labeled lymphocytes persist in the blood for the duration of infusions which lasted up to 220 days. It followed, then, that such lymphocytes must have been present before the infusion was started and therefore have a biologic life at least as long as the duration of the infusion. From the last observation it was concluded, there-

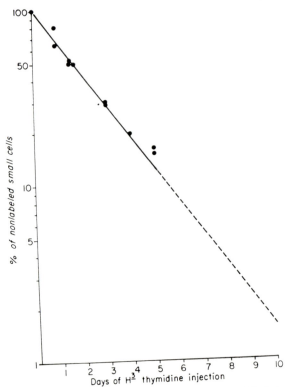

Figure 39. The rate of disappearance of nonlabeled small lymphocytes in the thymus after intramuscular injections of [3]HT. Note the linear rate of disappearance which suggests random departure. From Everett *et al.*[117]

fore, that the body does indeed contain a long-lived as well as a short-lived population of small lymphocytes, with the lifespan of the former being extremely long.[98-103,105-107,111,117,120]

Autoradiography was applied to lymphoid tissue sections to attempt to trace the sites of origin of short-lived and the elusive long-lived lymphocytes. The quantity (grains) of radioactivity acquired in lymphocytes of different lymphoid organs, different portions of lymphoid organs, and lymphocytes of different size were assessed at various time intervals following parenteral injections of [3]HT (see Fig. 38). By means of this technique, it was found that intense and early labeling appears in lymphocytes of the thymus and bone marrow, whereas moderately intense labeling appears simultaneously in the lymphocytes of the spleen.[98] In the peripheral lymph nodes, mesenteric lymph nodes and Peyer's patches examined at the same time after injection, the intensity of labeling appeared to be of a lower order.[98] Such findings seem to correlate well with the measurements on $^{32}PO_4$ incorporation into DNA per gram of tissue as found by Andreason and Ottesen.[113,114] They found through measuring DNA-^{32}P per gram of tissue 2 hours and 42 hours after injection of $^{32}PO_4$ in the rat that if over a period of time the newly formed labeled nucleic acid in the thymus is rated at 100, then lymph nodes of the lungs and skin equal 17.5, of spleen equal 16.3, of intestinal lymph nodes equal 15.6, and of Peyer's patches equal 10.5.

In the thymus, the intensity and rate of ^{3}HT labeling appeared most rapid in the large and medium-sized lymphocytes of the cortex, whereas in the remaining lymphoid tissues the most intense labeling occurred in some of the very large lymphocytes of the germinal centers and in the large and medium-sized lymphocytes of the primary follicles and more diffusely arranged lymphoid tissue.[16,23,55,98,121,122] In the concentrically arranged medium-sized lymphocytes surrounding the mantle zones of the secondary follicles, relatively uniform and intense labeling was found.[55,98,122] The densely packed small lymphocytes in the mantle zones and those in thymic medulla showed relatively little evidence of labeling.[16,55,122] In the thoracic duct, the intensely labeled cells, for the most part, proved to be medium-sized lymphocytes, many of which showed histologic evidence of active RNA synthesis in their cytoplasm.[98,104] Such data has been difficult for all to interpret, owing to the evidence of active lymphocyte production in all sites sampled, except the mantle zones immediately surrounding the germinal centers of the secondary lymph follicles. Here, many would expect to see relatively intense labeling, particularly if the very large precursor cells incorporating isotopes and dividing rapidly give rise to the surrounding compressed zone of very small lymphocytes.[55,101,122]

From these data, some researchers conclude that it is likely the rapidly growing small lymphocytes from the thymic cortex migrate in large numbers into the bloodstream and to the mantle zones of the lymph follicles to constitute a pool of slowly dividing, long-lived small lymphocytes whose purpose is to retain immunologic memory for prolonged periods. Other lymphocytes of shorter biologic life from the bursa of Fabricius (or its mammalian counterpart), or from the thymus (medulla?) may migrate to the paracortical areas of the spleen and nodes to transform there into antibody-producing cells. Such conclusions would seem to fit well with the data outlined above indicating that:

1. Lymphocytes are primarily concerned with immunity (sect. A).

2. They are long-lived cells destined to recirculate and colonize in other lymphoid tissues (sect. B).

3. They are cells capable of dedifferentiation and resumption of antibody synthesis (sect. C).

4. They are cells derived in relatively large numbers from thymic epithelium during embryonal life (sect. D).

Many people remain puzzled, however, by the numbers involved in each parameter and how these small, relatively nondescript cells actually acquire their specific immunologic attributes. Survey of recent hypotheses at home [24-26,98] and abroad [27,123,124] fail to reveal unanimous opinions, perhaps owing to the facts that

1. Mixtures of thymus cells and bone marrow cells (specific cell types unspecified) are more effective then thymus cells alone in conferring immunologic competence on animals rendered immunologically incompetent by total body irradiation.

2. A true counterpart to the bursa of Fabricius remains to be identified in mammals.

3. Relatively few persons consider that some thymus and bursal cells, particularly the epithelial cells, may exert a truely endocrine function, merely producing a hormone which accelerates the rate of DNA synthesis in cells nearby and more remotely located.

4. Cells which synthesize DNA relatively rapidly must utilize DNA precursors, DNA from other cells, or both in order to grow at a relatively rapid rate.

5. If DNA from other lymphoid or nonlymphoid cells is reutilized, its genetic code may be expressed in the recipient cells.

6. Other types of lymphoid cells, besides lymphocytes and plasmacytes, appear to be involved in immunologic responses.

2. The Basis for Counterarguments

The flaw in the interpretation of the isotopic data upon which recent concepts are based, lies not in tracing utilization of isotope labeled precursors, but in the failure to trace the utilization of unlabeled precursors which constitute the bulk of substrate from which DNA is actually synthesized during the period of experimental study. The precursors can come only from other cells or from food ingested. They do not ordinarily come from intramuscular or intravenous injections in healthy, free living individuals or in animals subjected to study for any extended period of time, e.g. 8 hours or more. To explain why the pattern of utilization of precursors may differ from lymphoid organ to lymphoid organ and why patterns differ in different portions of lymphoid organs, it is necessary to trace the ultimate origin and distribution of substrate from which DNA is ordinarily being synthesized.

Insofar as the ultimate origin of substrate is concerned, it must come from digested food once placental connections are disrupted. (See Sect. 3 for a detailed description of substrate utilization prior to birth.) The principal surface from which digested food is absorbed is the small intestine, through the mucosal cells of its villi. It is known that the lymphoid tissue of the lamina propria which supports the mucosal cells is poorly developed at birth.[74,125-128] However, as soon as the neonate commences to eat, the lymphoid tissue in the lamina propria grows very rapidly to constitute a mass of relatively diffuse and nodular lymphoid tissue whose total mass approaches that of the spleen.[127,128] Each time the individual ingests a meal containing

of DNA precursor incorporation.[98-110] This would seem to indicate that the lymphoid tissues grow relatively rapidly in comparison with remaining tissues in the body. However, both by the single (flash) injection and the continuous infusion techniques it has been found, despite rapid and intense nuclear labeling in many lymphocytes, nuclear labeling fails to occur in other morphologically similar cells, irrespective of the time of sampling. While the latter findings are currently explained by postulating the coexistence of a rapidly growing, short-lived lymphocyte population and a morphologically similar, very slow growing, long-lived, functionally different population, there is another explanation.

b. Competitive Interference, Growth Rate, and Life Span Calculations

The thymus, bone marrow, and spleen differ from the nodes and the intestinal lymphoid tissue in that the former receive unlabeled (endogenous) and labeled (exogenous) DNA precursors entirely via afferent arteries, whereas the latter receive them not only from arteries but also via peripheral lymphatics (in the case of the nodes) or quite directly from mucosal cells concerned with absorption (in the case of intestinal lymphoid tissue). If the cells growing in nodes and those growing in the lamina propria of the small intestine utilize quantities of unlabeled DNA precursors from such additional sources, local situations will occur wherein there is increased competition with labeled precursors for positions in DNA being synthesized at the time of sampling. On the basis of favorable balance of unlabeled over labeled DNA precursors while competing for positions, one may explain relatively scant labeling of some lymphoid cells in the nodes, the intestinal lymphoid tissue, the thoracic duct lymph, and ultimately in the circulating blood.

The most obvious locus for competitive interference to take place, of course, is in the lymphoid tissue of the intestinal submucosa. Here lies the first opportunity for competition between parenterally injected, labeled DNA precursors and natural, unlabeled, chemically similar DNA precursors newly absorbed from food. As shown by Andreason and Ottesen,[113,114] the rate of labeling with injected $^{32}PO_4$ is slowest here. Unlabeled DNA precursors, such as natural phosphates (essential to growth in many parts of the body), are normally absorbed via adjacent mucosal cells. Immediately beneath the mucosal cells, lymphoid cells undergo inordinately rapid division [129] and increase in aggregate mass [128-130] during the absorption of a meal containing protein. From this submucosal lymphoid tissue and from the mesenteric nodes emanate the bulk of the lymphocytes to be found in thoracic duct lymph, particularly when the animal is feeding.[74,128-130] This explains two things. First, at time intervals greater than 24 hours after the parenteral injection of labeled DNA precursors (the humans or experimental animals meanwhile continuing to feed on their standard diets), unlabeled or poorly labeled lymphocytes are found in greater concentration in thoracic duct lymph than in circulating blood. Second, is explained why 100 days or more following the continuous intravenous infusion of labeled DNA precursors (the experimental animals continuing to maintain weight and survive on their standard diets) unlabeled or poorly labeled lymphocytes are found in thoracic duct lymph and circulating blood in very significant percentage. In other words, for as long as the individual continues to eat and absorb more unlabeled DNA precursors via the intestine, such precursors will compete successfully with parenterally injected labeled precursors to the extent that all proliferating lymphocytes (and other cells) in the body can become intensely labeled, before a comparable level of labeling will be evident in the absorptive cells of the intestinal villi, the lymphoid cells which grow underneath them, and the lymphocytes which migrate from there into the thoracic duct on their way to the circulating bloodstream.

Somewhat less obvious is the situation in the lymph nodes. Via their afferent arteries and their afferent lymphatics they normally receive unlabeled DNA precursors and continue to receive them after the injection of a given labeled DNA precursor. After injection, irrespective of the molecular weight of the given DNA precursor, its concentration or ratio with respect to chemically

similar circulating endogenous DNA precursors will become uniform throughout the blood vascular system within minutes owing
to the rapidity and efficiency with which mixing takes place
there). Within minutes or hours, depending on the molecular
weight (hence diffusing capacity) of the given precursor, its ratio
or concentration with respect to similar unlabeled precursors will
become uniform throughout the body fluids, including lymph,
interstitial fluid, and intracellular fluid. Theoretically, therefore,
all cells in the body will have equal opportunity to utilize the
labeled precursor, instead of its natural counterpart.

Having utilized the labeled precursor (along with its naturally
occurring, chemically similar counterpart) at rates which reflect
the rate of protoplasmic growth from all precursors, the cells may
release the precursors at rates commensurate with their life span.
However, they may do so in forms which are more complex than
the original simple precursors. Precursors residing in compounds
of relatively high molecular weight which do not diffuse readily
generally return to the regional lymph nodes via the peripheral
or afferent nodal lymphatics. Therefore, in afferent nodal lymph,
one may expect to find DNA precursors which have diffused from
the arteriovenous circulation but which are diluted into a solution containing chemically similar precursors returning from
peripheral tissue cells in simple or complex forms. Moreover, one
may expect to find a relatively high percentage of returning unlabeled precursors which were synthesized into peripheral cell
protoplasm before the given labeled precursor was injected. Diluted into an unknown volume of simple and more complex
precursors, the ratio or concentration of the given labeled precursor, accordingly, may be reduced in afferent nodal lymph. As
a result, the regional nodes (especially their medullary portions)
may show an unexpectedly low order of cell labeling owing to a
relatively high concentration of unlabeled precursors. On these
grounds, one may explain the relatively low order of cell labeling
in lymph nodes generally. (It is important to recall here that
utilizing $^{32}PO_4$ as the label, Andreason and Ottesen [113-114] calculated labeling indices as follows: thymus, 100; nodes regional to

lungs and skin, 17.5; spleen 16.3; intestinal lymph nodes, 15.6; and Peyer's patches, 10.5.)

The mesenteric nodes are outstanding among the nodes in which to search for this form of competitive interference. Relatively rich in newly absorbed, unlabeled DNA precursors, simple or complex (as compared with circulating blood) the intestinal lymph drains into the mesenteric nodes and is filtered there before flowing onward to constitute the bulk of the lymph in the thoracic duct. Within the mesenteric nodes, relatively high concentrations of newly absorbed, unlabeled precursors (whether they be simple or attached to other larger molecules) upon entering with intestinal lymph, may compete favorably with injected labeled similar DNA precursors brought in via the arterial circulation. As a result, DNA-synthesizing cells in the mesenteric nodes (especially the cells in medullary portions) may show a relatively low order of labeling. (It is pertinent to add here that the mesenteric nodes are unique in that they are regional not only to parenchymal cells concerned with absorption but also to a cell population whose calculated life span is almost as short as that of most, if not all, lymphocytes.)

In the spleen, periarteriolar lymphoid tissue of the marrow, and thymus competetive interference between injected, isotope labeled, and newly absorbed, unlabeled, DNA precursors (or unlabeled precursors emanating from peripheral tissue cells), at first glance, would seem negligible. This is owing to the fact that the spleen, periarteriolar lymphoid tissue of the marrow, and thymus lack a nearby nonlymphoid cellular source of unlabeled DNA precursors; they lack afferent lymphatics; and they are supplied with DNA precursors entirely via their afferent arteries. The thoracic duct lymph which emanates largely from the intestine and mesenteric nodes, upon flowing into the systemic arteriovenous circulation, mixes so rapidly that ratios between labeled and unlabeled DNA precursors become quite uniform, irrespective of where arterial or systemic venous blood are sampled. In order to explain why labeling patterns differ in these arterially fed segments of the lymphoid tissue mass, one must look toward variations in arterial circulation during absorption, and toward local factors which accelerate DNA synthesis.

The spleen differs from the periarteriolar lymphoid tissue of the marrow in that its arterial blood supply is relatively large (e.g. 2 L per minute,[286] as compared with a resting cardiac output of 5 L per minute) and that its arterial flow rate increases during absorption, along with that in the entire splanchnic vascular bed.[131] On the other hand, the arterial supply of the marrow appears relatively small and has not been observed to increase during absorption. Moreover, if arterial flow during absorption is largely directed toward the splanchnic vascular bed, the arterial supply of the marrow may be correspondingly decreased. Increased arterial flow during absorption assures the splenic receipt of a relatively large share of unlabeled DNA precursors entering the blood circulation via thoracic duct lymph (incidentally, produced in relatively large quantities by intestinal and mesenteric lymphoid tissues during absorption). Therefore, on the basis of flooding with relatively large quantities of unlabeled DNA precursors during absorption, one may explain a relatively low uptake of injected, labeled DNA precursors in the spleen, as compared with the periarteriolar lymphoid tissue of the marrow.

The thymus resembles the periarteriolar lymphoid tissue of the marrow and differs from the spleen in that it is entirely supplied by systemic arteries other than those supplying the splanchnic vascular bed within the peritoneal cavity. (To what extent the systemic arterial supply increases within the throracic cavity and lower neck during absorption is not clear, even though pulmonary arterial flow increases to some extent.) Moreover, the thymus differs from the periarteriolar lymphoid tissue of the bone marrow, the spleen, and all remaining segments of the lymphoid tissue mass in that its lymphoid cells grow in intimate relation with epithelial cells specialized to produce a hormone which accelerates DNA synthesis in lymphocytes (see Chap. 15). Thus, relatively lacking in competitive interference from newly absorbed, unlabeled DNA precursors and lying next to the cellular source of a hormone which accelerates DNA synthesis, one may explain why the lymphoid cells of the thymus incorporate relatively large quantities of injected, labeled DNA precursors and appear to grow at an extremely high rate.

In conclusion, then, through competitive interference between newly absorbed, unlabeled DNA precursors and injected isotope labeled identical compounds and analysis of how the former move from points of absorption, while the latter circulate after injection, one may explain these three points:

1. Why the thymus, periarteriolar lymphoid tissue of the marrow, spleen, intestinal lymph nodes, and submucosal lymphoid tissue of the small intestine show decremental orders of labeling with isotope-labeled DNA precursors (see the $^{32}PO_4$ labeling indices of Andreason and Ottesen alluded to earlier and Dr. Everett's observations with the use of injected tritiated thymidine, Fig. 38).

2. Why some of the aforementioned segments of the lymphoid tissue mass are calculated to synthesize DNA and grow much more rapidly than others when they are not necessarily doing so.

3. Why some circulating lymphocytes (particularly those which emanate from the intestine and its mesentery), failing to become labeled with parenterally injected, isotope-labeled DNA precursors are not necessarily cells of very prolonged biologic life.

Such explanations might be particularly helpful to those used to studying the lymphoid organs from clinical, histologic, or physiologic points of view and who wonder why labeling patterns seem to correlate poorly with clinical observations, catheterization data,[74,128] mitotic indices,[141,142] and DNA-bound phosphorous determinations (see Tables VI–VIII). The latter have all supplied useful and heretofore reliable estimates of relative growth rates and life spans in various kinds of lymphoid, as well as non-lymphoid, cells. Morever, such explanations may put an end to the cacophony of lymphocyte migration streams and homing predilections currently postulated by experimental biologists more concerned with the fate of injected isotope labeled DNA precursors than with the sources from which lymphocytes actually obtain the substrate essential to growth.

c. Reutilization and Recirculation

The foregoing considerations remain to be digested by the more casual reader and recognized as valid by the more expert, but current consensus holds, on the basis of the data outlined above, that the lymphoid organ, lymph, and circulating blood contain at least two lymphocyte populations. One is calculated to be of short biologic life (e.g. 24 to 48 hours), while the other is calculated to be of biologic life ranging from two days to many years.

As already mentioned, the existence, but indefinite life span of the latter population has been predicted on the basis of two types of isotope experiments. First, there were experiments showing that unlabeled lymphocytes persist in thoracic duct lymph and circulating blood for periods of time longer than the duration of continuous parenteral infusions with isotope labeled DNA precursors. The assumption here is that these particular unlabeled calls must have been present in the body before the infusion was started and therefore must be of a longer biologic life than the duration of the infusion. Second, there were experiments showing that after single or multiple parenteral injections of isotope-labeled DNA precursors, it takes a very long time for all labeled lymphocytes to disappear from thoracic duct lymph and circulating blood. The assumption here is that these particular labeled cells enjoy prolonged biologic life. Having dealt with the "persistence of unlabeled lymphocytes" in the previous section, issue will be taken here with current interpretations of the data on labeled ones.

Theoretically, as compared with other cell populations, a cell population which grows very rapidly and therefore is of short biologic life will not only utilize injected labeled DNA precursors rapidly but also (if not excreted from the body) reutilize labeled DNA from its own short-lived cells at a rapid rate. Noting the lack of secondary peaks in disappearance curves of labeled lymphocytes and pointing to the declining exponential form of these curves, Trowell [118] and Hamilton [119] were among the first to suggest that quantitatively important reutilization of isotope-labeled DNA precursors takes place in the lymphoid organs, with the DNA from relatively large numbers of circulating lymphocytes being reutilized in the neoformation of others. Considerable immunologic significance was accorded to this interpretation of the data (see above and Chap. 18).

Good histologic and physiologic evidence supports the reutilization hypothesis of Trowell and Hamilton. Lymphocytopoieis, as judged by mitotic indices, appears extremely active in lymphoid organs where relatively large numbers of lymphocytes are disintegrating, as in the thymus, spleen, lymph nodes, and Peyer's patches.[16,141,142] The only notable exception is in the bone marrow, where lymphocyte mitoses appear rare,[141,142] but labeling with DNA precursors is relatively great (see Fig. 38). Data obtained by lymphatic catheterization indicate that for every lymphocyte which enters the afferent lymphatics of a node, 30 leave via the efferent lymphatics.[115] Sufficient lymphocytes are delivered via the thoracic duct into the circulating blood to completely replace the circulating blood lymphocyte population 2 to 12 times daily (depending on the species studied).[115] Figures of 8 times daily (every three hours) have been given for rats and 6 times daily (every four hours) for humans.[115] Such figures, however, may be subject to variation, depending on thoracic duct output as a function of diet.[74,127,128] Moreover, relatively short instead of prolonged biologic life of lymphocytes in general is indicated by comparative studies on DNA-bound phosphorous (DNA-P) in various tissues (see Tables VI–VIII) and measurements of the rate of DNA-^{32}P turnover [115] which reflect the actual rate at which DNA is synthesized in various tissues.

Two loopholes in the reutilization hypothesis have become evident, however. The first (to be considered later, on pp. 187-201.) is that although lymphocyte disintegration is very obvious in the germinal centers of many lymphoid organs, the germinal centers do not appear to give rise to the densely packed small lymphocytes in the mantle zones which immediately surround them.[55] The second is that the persistence of a long-lived population of

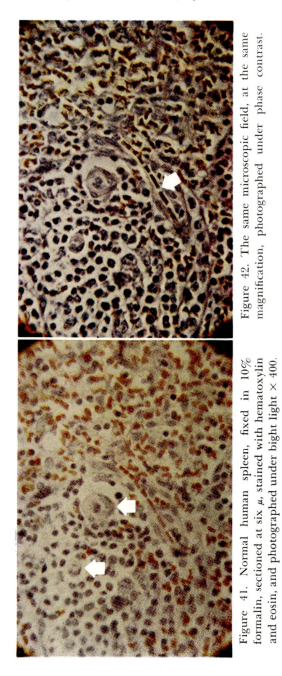

Figure 42. The same microscopic field, at the same magnification, photographed under phase contrast.

Figure 41. Normal human spleen, fixed in 10% formalin, sectioned at six μ, stained with hematoxylin and eosin, and photographed under bright light × 400.

Figures 41 and 42. Note the following:

1. The relative absence of erythrocytes in the periarteriolar lymphoid tissue surrounding two small muscular arterioles cut in cross section.

2. The compressed appearance of the relatively few erythrocytes lying between medium-sized and small lymphocytes in the periarteriolar lymphoid tissue, and the lack of visible vascular structures containing the erythrocytes.

3. The compression and elongation of the row of erythrocytes in the ellipsoid (arrow) emerging tangentially from the periarteriolar lymphoid tissue.

4. The relative lack of compression of the many erythrocytes in the pulp spaces below and to the right of the ellipsoid.

5. How phase contrast accentuates the fibrillar content of the reticulum in which the arterioles and the lymphocytes are supported.

←———

ever, the situation is very different and as superlative as the incredible motility of the small lymphocyte.

For descriptions of the circulation in lymphoid organs, we are particularly indebted to Weidenreich,[154] Jaeger,[155] and Maximow,[156] who studied the problem in serial histologic sections, and to Knisely[157] and MacKenzie,[131] who described the circulation of the living spleen as it appears under transillumination at high magnifications. Lucid descriptions of the circulation in relation to the stroma and cells are to be found in communications by the late Drs. Klemperer,[37] Jaffé,[38] and Ehrich.[158]

The crux of the problem, insofar as the ordinary microscopist is concerned, is that lymphoid organs are primarily arterial organs, normally perfused under a head of mean arterial pressure in excess of 80 mm Hg. When the afferent artery or arteries are ligated and this head of pressure is cut off in the lymphoid organ or organs selected for histologic study, the elastic recoil of the arterial muscularis and the surrounding elastic stroma is so powerful that the blood becomes distributed distally along the lines of least resistance.[131] As a result, the white pulp of the spleen, the periarteriolar lymphoid tissue of the marrow, and the cortex of the lymph nodes usually appear quite bloodless. Careful scrutiny, however, will still reveal erythrocytes singly or in rows, lying in a highly compressed condition within the reticulum which supports the growing lymphocytes (see Figs. 41 and 42). Therefore, in order to assess what transpires during life, one must rely on more than one method of study and draw conclusions which may seem arbitrary, particularly with respect to the long-standing argument concerning whether the arterial circulation is open or closed, i.e. lined or unlined by endothelium.[37,131,157]

In my opinion,* there is essentially no difference between the arterial circulation in the white pulp of the spleen, in the cortex of the remaining lymphoid organs, in the periarteriolar lymphoid tissue of normal bone marrow and in the nodular lymphoid tissue of the intestine. As pointed out by Ehrich,[158] all of these areas contain arterioles but no true veins or lymphatics. Description, therefore, can be greatly simplified (as is Fig. 1). The arterioles appear relatively large in caliber in comparison with the mass of tissue they are destined to supply, as they leave the fibrous or bony septa to enter nodular masses of growing lymphocytes (see Figs. 43–45). As they enter the nodules, the muscular arterioles give off many tiny arcuate (arched) branches devoid of muscle tunics, which soon become devoid of endothelium. In such branches, the blood is contained only by the reticulum which

---

* This opinion is based on the following:

1. Personal study of serial histologic sections of human spleen, lymph nodes, and marrow under phase, as well as ordinary light microscopy (see Table I and references 48, 145, 146, and 150 for material studied). Phase microscopy seemed particularly helpful in studying relations of fibrils to cells in H & E sections, not visible under ordinary light microscopy (see Fig. 42). Simultaneous study of unsectioned tissue fragments obtained from the same organs by the needle aspiration technique seem particularly helpful in that the third dimension becomes more apparent in studying relationships between reticulum, endothelium, and non-motile elements from the circulation, such as erythrocytes and thrombocytes.

2. Review of the older literature, particularly as summarized by Klemperer,[37] in which it was observed and concluded by several (including Ecker, Leydig, Stieda, Mueller, Henle, Kultschitzky, Gray, Hoyer, and Weidenreich) that an open, as well as a closed, arterial circulation is demonstrable in lymphoid organs.

3. Review of descriptions of microcirculation in living transilluminated spleens by Mackenzie [131] and photographed by Whipple *et al.*,[159] who concluded that an open, as well as a closed, arterial circulation is demonstrable; the former being open intermittently, and open only when relatively normal levels of arterial blood pressure and arterial oxygenation were maintained; whereas the latter, closed circulation, carried flowing blood more or less constantly, even when arterial pressure and oxygenation were reduced.

4. The consideration that an intermittently open circulation not only allows for the flow of nonmotile macromolecules and formed elements produced in hematopoietic organs into the systemic blood and lymph circulation but also makes allowance for the flow of circulating elements back into the hematopoietic organs so that they can be reutilized in myelopoieis and lymphopoiesis (see Sect. 3).

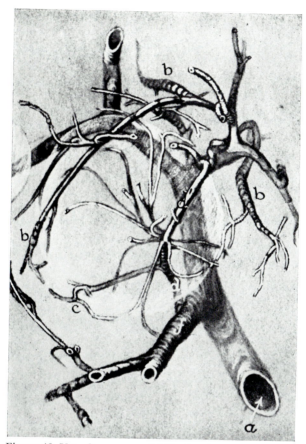

Figure 43. Vascular system of fully developed malpighian corpuscle. Graphic reconstruction from serial sections. Magnification × 70. Uppermost sections with part of surrounding sheathed arteries have been omitted for clear demonstration of internal vascular network. a, Follicular artery; b, sheathed penicilliary artery; c, "Hof" artery; d, arterial loop of internal net; f, point of origin of second limb of arterial loop behind large vessels (not visible). (Courtesy of Dr. E. Jaeger, 1929.) From Klemperer, P.[37]

contains concentrically oriented, tightly packed small and medium-sized lymphocytes. (Such arcuate branches are described by Jaeger[155] within the lymph follicles, and as observed by

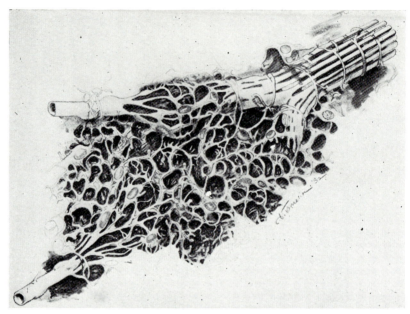

Figure 44. Semidiagrammatic drawing of intermediary circulation of human spleen. This drawing represents Dr. Klemperer's concept of the architecture of the reticulum and its relation to finest blood channels. Although it is not an actual reconstruction of serial sections, all structural details which are depicted in three dimensions have been observed histologically. For technical reasons, reticular fibers have not been drawn in different color but as ridges upon cytoplasmic syncytium. From Klemperer, P.[37]

MacKenzie,[131] the blood flows through them at a very rapid rate but intermittently.)

In the secondary lymph follicles, which usually lie close to the points where the arterials emerge from the septa, the large afferent muscular arteriole usually gives off a tiny capillary which courses in an irregular manner through the germinal center. In the middle of the germinal center, the capillary endothelium resembles sinusoidal endothelium and the surrounding cells resemble the syncytial reticulum or "active mesenchyme" found in the red pulp of the spleen (cf. Klemperer[37] and Jaffé[38]). The architecture of the germinal center (with relatively undifferentiated reticular stroma, a tiny primitive vessel, and variable numbers of large, deeply basophilic cells) is remindful of an island

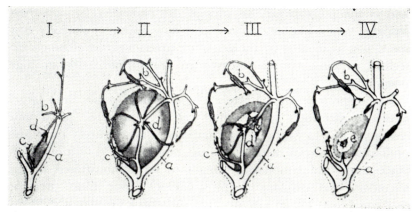

Figure 45. Vessels of malp'ghian corpuscles during involution phases. I, follicle formation. II, follicle with developed internal net. III, involution with hyaline deposits upon internal net. IV, transition into resting stage with loss of internal net. a, follicular artery; b, sheathed artery (penicillus); c, "Hof" artery; d, internal net; e, hyaline deposits. (Courtesy of Dr. E. Jaeger, 1929.) From Klemperer, P.[37]

of primitive yolk sac mesenchyme or an island of splenic red pulp but an island stranded proximally beside a relatively large (eccentric) arteriole. Differing from the embryonal mesenchyme and the splenic red pulp, the germinal center island is surrounded by regular monotonous rows of densely packed, compressed small lymphocytes between which arterial blood flows rapidly but intermittently in arcuate (arch-like) channels.

In the primary lymph follicles located distal to the secondary lymph follicles along the course of arterial supply, the muscular arterioles give off more arcuate branches between concentric rows of medium-sized and small lymphocytes of slightly less compressed appearance than those surrounding germinal centers. After giving off the germinal center capillary and arcuate branches already mentioned, the main (or thoroughfare) portions of the arterioles pursue straight (pencil-like) courses toward the medullary portions of the spleen and nodes to terminate in bulbous structures lacking muscular tunics and having relatively thick endothelium reminiscent of sinusoidal endothelium. These bulbous structures probably correspond to what are described as the clubbed or pulp arterioles which feed the splenic ellipsoids,[37]

such as phosphate or thymidine, are labeled with radioactive isotopes, their initial utilization and their reutilization following incorporation into given cell types should parallel and be identical with the pathways followed by natural precursors. The isotope label merely offers a convenient method of recognizing where DNA is ordinarily being synthesized or reutilized at given points in time after its introduction into the body's pool of similar unlabeled precursors. A relatively rich arterial circulation in lymphoid organs provides growing lymphoid cells with an initial opportunity to utilize relatively large quantities of labeled, as well as unlabeled, DNA precursors, whereas an intermittently open circulation through portions of the reticulum provides an opportuntity for subsequent reutilization of relatively large quantities of labeled, as well as unlabeled, DNA precursors incorporated previously within other cells which normally circulate.

vi. THE CIRCULATION RELATED TO THE ISOTOPE DATA. Assuming that injected, isotope-labeled and endogenous, unlabeled DNA precursors have been incorporated into lymphocytes growing in various lymphoid organs, it must be assumed further that they will be released to become available to other growing cells (irrespective of kind) in the following order. As precursors bound to cells, many of which are actively motile, and many of which circulate; as precursors bound to proteins emanating from intact and degenerating cells, many of which will circulate; and as free precursors, many of which will circulate and which will diffuse more rapidly than the precursors bound to free extracellular proteins. Of such forms, only the precursors bound to intact cells or to cells in early stages of disintegration will be relatively easy to trace during passage from one cell to another in the same organ or from the cells of one organ to another via the circulation.

Review of the ³HT data already presented will reveal the following facts. 1. After single, spaced, or continuous infusion of the labeled DNA precursor, the rate of labeling prior to, during, and after peak labeling is greatest in large, relatively great in medium-sized, and least in small lymphocytes.[55,98-107] 2. At the same time, in each lymphoid organ studied, labeling will appear greatest in the medullary (paracortical) areas, lesser in the primary follicles, and least in the secondary follicles [55,98,117,121,122] (owing to the fact that the medullary areas contain the least, the primary follicles contain a higher, and the secondary follicles contain the highest proportion of small lymphocytes). Such findings indicate that the rate of reutilization of labeled and unlabeled precursors in given types of cells and in given portions of lymphoid organs closely parallel the initial rates of incorporation of the precursors and that the bulk of reutilization takes place in portions of the lymphoid organs and in those types of cells wherein the rates of initial incorporation are the highest. Therefore, one must look toward the large and medium-sized lymphocytes as the potential recipients of unlabeled and labeled precursors carried primarily by unlabeled and labeled cells (or their products) which originate in various lymphoid organs and actually circulate from one organ to another or which circulate from one portion of a given lymphoid organ to another portion.

The observations that unlabeled and labeled small lymphocytes normally appear to migrate through the endothelium of the bulbous arterioles (or postcapillary venules) of some lymphoid organs,[72] that arterial blood flow remains relatively constant through these terminal branches of (straight) thoroughfare arterioles,[131,157] and that a large share of the reutilization of [3]HT-labeled DNA precursors takes place in the medullary reticulum where they terminate [55,98,117,121,122] all suggest that a relatively large proportion of circulating blood lymphocytes give up their DNA to be reutilized in the medium-sized lymphocytes which constitute the bulk of cells in the medullary reticulum of various lymphoid organs. Moreover, because there is minimal evidence of phagocytosis of small lymphocyte nuclei in the perifollicular (paracortical) reticulum where the bulbous arterioles terminate,[141,142,147] it must be assumed that the small lymphocytes emanating from the arteriolar blood give up their DNA (containing unlabeled and labeled precursors) more or less directly to the rapidly proliferating, short-lived, medium-sized lymphocytes which differentiate heteroplastically from the medullary reticulum.[147] Such an assumption is enhanced by the fact that careful scrutiny in imprints and sections will reveal that many of the free lymphocytes in the medullary areas of the spleen, nodes, and marrow have bare nuclei showing diffuse chromotalysis and absence of surrounding cytoplasm [147,163]—signs of degeneration and disintegration. The assumption is enhanced further by the observation that karyotype-labeling studies *in vivo* (see Chap. 16) are compatible with, and suggestive of, reutilization of emigrating small-lymphocyte DNA in the form of intact molecules and within a relatively short period of time (e.g. 12 hours). The assumption is enhanced also by the fact that mammalian cells *in vitro* may incorporate DNA from viruses or from other human cells and proceed to demonstrate altered genotypic characteristics (see Chap. 16, B,C).

An almost diametrically opposite situation from the medullary areas of most lymphoid organs is to be found in the germinal centers of the secondary lymph follicles and in the cortex of the thymus. Whereas the germinal centers and the thymic cortex lack an obviously rich (and continuous) arterial blood supply, both incorporate and reutilize unlabeled as well as labeled nuclear material at rates which would seem to be quite rapid.[16,55,98,121,122] While a rapid rate of incorporation of DNA precursors and a rapid rate of reutilization of such precursors can be explained in the thymic cortex on the basis of local production of a hormone which accelerates DNA synthesis into lymphocytes locally produced,[96] such an explanation would not seem to suffice in the germinal centers.

Close scrutiny of the thymic cortex and the germinal centers will reveal that both contain relatively large numbers of disintegrating lymphocyte nuclei (tingible bodies) to be found within Hassall's corpuscles of the thymus [164,165] and in histiocytic components of the reticulum in the germinal centers.[29,141,142,147] In contrast to the diffuse chromatolysis of disintegrating lymphocyte nuclei in the medullary areas, nuclear remnants in Hassall's corpuscles and in the histiocytes of the germinal centers appear to undergo disintegration by nuclear pyknosis and fragmentation and appear to be digested there. In the thymic cortex radiating out from the nuclear graveyard in the Hassall's corpuscles, the corpuscular cytoplasm peels off like the rings of an onion and fades imperceptibly into the syncytial cytoplasm of the adjacent epithelial reticular cells and onward into the mesenchymal reticulum where large lymphocytes appear to differentiate from mesenchymal reticular cells.[95,164] On the other hand, in the germinal centers radiating out from the disintegrating nuclei of small lymphocytes and other debris within the histiocytic components of the reticulum, the syncytial cytoplasm of the histiocytes fades imperceptibly on into the reticulum where large lymphocytes appear to differentiate from similar mesenchymal reticular cells.[147]

To recapitulate and continue, then, it would seem that a relatively rich, open arterial circulation in the medullary (paracortical) reticulum and a relative lack of it in the epithelial portion of the thymic cortex and in the germinal centers play a significant role in the pattern of reutilization of migratory lymphocytes, along with other substances necessary for growth. For instance, in the medullary reticulum, the circulation appears such that growing cells are bathed directly in arterial blood which flows relatively constantly from throughfare (straight) arterioles and bathed directly in arterial blood which flows intermittently via open, arcuate channels into the medullary reticulum. As a result of relatively great overall arterial flow rates via both types of arterial channels, growing cells in the medullary (paracortical) reticulum reside in a position to utilize (or reutilize) relatively large quantities of (a) labeled lymphocytes, unlabeled lymphocytes, labeled DNA precursors, unlabeled DNA precursors, and many other forms of substrate from circulating arterial blood, such as oxygen, glucose, amino acids, fats, etc., and (b) all of the substances mentioned in (a), together with cells or cellular products produced in the follicular reticulum, but flushed onward into the medullary reticulum by the arterial blood which flows intermittently through the follicular reticulum (via the arcuate channels). Quantitatively great utilization (or reutilization) of the former (a) is reflected directly in the rapid rate of utilization (or reutilization) of isotope-labeled DNA precursors, such as ^{3}HT—whether it be in the form of free precursor or in the form of precursor bound to the DNA of small circulating lymphocytes.

Quantitatively great reutilization of lymphocytes or cell products normally produced in the follicular reticulum is not obvious in [3]HT studies under normal conditions when the individual is feeding, and the rate of lymphoid cell birth and cell death are in equilibrium. However, reutilization may be reflected during starvation when the small lymphocyte population in the follicles disappears more rapidly than the medium-sized lymphocyte population in the medullary (paracortical) reticulum. Reutilization becomes quite obvious during more acute forms of stress when the follicular lymphocytes undergo rapid cytolysis, while medullary lymphoid cells show increased ingestion and phagocytosis of disintegrating nuclear material.[12,56]

Within the epithelial reticulum of the thymic cortex, where blood circulation is entirely lacking,[16,164] it would appear that the epithelial reticular cells digest relatively small numbers of pyknotic nuclear fragments from migrating small lymphocytes which have penetrated to Hassall's corpuscles[165] by virtue of their own independent (random) motility. While arterioles are present in the lymphoid tissue which surrounds the epithelial reticular cells containing the Hassall's corpuscles, the distance from arterioles to the epithelial cells and the Hassall's corpuscles is relatively large, as compared with the distance from arterioles to growing lymphoid cells. Therefore, it would appear that the epithelial reticular cells and the Hassall's corpuscles which they contain reside in a position where they may utilize (or reutilize) limited quantities of substances carried in arterial blood (as compared with the lymphoid tissue proper), as is evidenced by a low rate of incorporation of [3]HT in the epithelial reticular cells, as compared with lymphoid cells.[16,98,121]

In the reticulum of the germinal centers, each of which usually contains a very small capillary, it would appear that the majority of small lymphocytes and other large molecules which can be traced directly, such as nuclei of other types of cells, acid colloidal dyes, and foreign proteins, are utilized (or reutilized) in histiocytes adjacent to the capillaries.[37,38,147] As these capillaries are relatively small in comparison with the volume of germinal center reticulum which surrounds them, it would appear further that the mesenchymal reticulum of the germinal centers, like the epithelial reticulum of the thymus, is poorly supplied with substrate essential to cell growth, as compared with the medullary (paracortical) reticulum. The relative lack of substrate, again, may be evidenced in a relatively low rate of direct incorporation of [3]HT in the mesenchymal reticulum of the germinal centers, despite a functional capacity to grow and differentiate rapidly.[55,98,122]

In the medullary (paracortical) reticulum of lymphoid organs where arterial circulation appears relatively rich and open, disintegrating nuclear substance of migrating small lymphocytes may be reutilized *directly* by mesenchymal reticular cells and the medium-sized lymphocytes into which the former differentiate. On the other hand, in the epithelial portion of the thymic cortex and in the germinal centers, where circulation is lacking or appears relatively poor, respectively, the ingested pyknotic nuclear substance of migrating small lymphocytes may be reutilized in thymic epithelial reticular cells or in germinal center histiocytes which digest the nuclear substance before passing it on to adjacent mesenchymal reticular cells which subsequently differentiate into large lymphocytes (or other types of cells).[22,29,34,36-38,54,156]

In other words, the mesenchymal reticular cells and their medium-sized lymphocyte (or plasmacyte) progeny in the medullary reticulum are situated in such a way that they may *directly* reutilize relatively large quantities of substance, particularly DNA, of lymphocytes carried in by a relatively rich, open afferent arterial circulation. In contrast, the mesenchymal reticular cells and their progeny in the thymic cortex and in the germinal centers are so situated that they may reutilize relatively small quantities of substance, particularly DNA, of small lymphocytes which migrate from a poor arterial circulation, and do so *indirectly,* i.e. after previous digestion of this substance in adjacent epithelial reticular cells and histiocytes, respectively. Moreover, being integral components of a mesenchymal or reticular syncytium (according to Downey [147] and others [33,38]), dividing without mitosis (according to several researchers [33,34,145]), and showing little, if any, direct incorporation of the labeled DNA

precursor, [3]HT,[98,121,122] it would appear that the nuclei of mesenchymal reticular cells are *obliged* to reutilize substances,
particularly DNA, from disintegrating nuclei in the medullary
reticulum and from predigested cells in the thymic cortex and
germinal centers in order to differentiate and grow into the various types of cells found in these areas normally, as well as under
experimental or abnormal conditions.

In summary and conclusion, then, it would appear from this
interpretation of the data on the arterial circulation in lymphoid
organs, as it related to the utilization and reutilization of DNA
precursors, that the following is important.

1. Within the medullary reticulum of lymphoid organs, a
rich, open arterial circulation not only enables great, direct
utilization of simple labeled and unlabeled DNA precursors,
along with other circulating substances (such as oxygen, glucose,
amino acids, fats, etc.), but also enables great direct reutilization
of labeled and unlabeled DNA and other complex substances
from disintegrating lymphocytes emanating from other lymphoid
organs and carried in via the systemic arterial circulation or
emanating from another portion of the same lymphoid organ
and carried into the medullary reticulum via the organ's own
open arterial circulation. Thus great direct utilization of the
former simple precursors would appear to be essential to the
production of relatively great quantities of lymphoid cells and
plasma in the medullary (paracortical) reticulum of not one,
but many, lymphoid organs. At the same time, great direct
reutilization of DNA and other complex substances from circulating lymphocytes may serve to determine the quality of lymphoid cells and plasma produced there.

2. Within the epithelial reticulum of the thymic cortex, a lack of
arterial circulation precludes massive utilization of the former
relatively simple substances outlined above but does not preclude
reutilization of substances such as DNA from the relatively small
number of lymphocytes which happen to migrate independently
into the epithelial reticular cells. The thymic epithelial reticular
cells, then, may utilize the pyknotic nuclei of degenerating migratory lymphocytes along with their own pyknotic nuclei and

relatively small quantities of simple precursors which diffuse from a relatively distant and locally poor arterial circulation. A hormone may be produced from all this which accelerates DNA synthesis (and lymphocytopoiesis) in the surrounding mesenchymal reticulum. Finally, the small number of lymphocytes which happen to migrate into and degenerate within the Hassall's corpuscles (possibly by feeding back) may regulate, first, the rate of hormone production in the thymic epithelial reticular cells; second, the rate of lymphocytopoiesis in the thymus; and third, the rate of lymphopoiesis throughout the lymphoid organs (cf. Chap. 15).

3. Within the germinal centers a relatively small capillary circulation limits the availability of substrate in general but does not limit the reutilization of substance, particularly DNA, of those lymphocytes which happen to migrate at random from the small germinal center capillaries into the surrounding mesenchymal reticulum. The histiocytic components of the mesenchymal reticulum surrounding the capillary in order to furnish digested substrate to adjacent undifferentiated mesenchymal reticular cells then may reutilize the pyknotic nuclei of some of the emigrating lymphocytes, along with other nuclear and cellular debris, and free extracellular proteins from other cells (or microorganisms) and small quantities of simple substances which diffuse from the tiny capillary. The histiocytic feedback and subsequent reutilization of such digested substrate within the mesenchymal reticular cells of the germinal centers, then, may serve to determine the quality of subsequent lymphopoiesis, first in the germinal centers and later, in the surrounding follicular reticulum—not just in one lymphoid organ, but in many (see ensuing section on germinal centers). Moreover, because the germinal center histiocytes appear to incorporate nuclei and cellular debris from other types of cells, free extracellular proteins of exogenous, endogenous, or microbial origin, as well as the pyknotic nuclei of lymphocytes, it must be presumed that all are potential determinants of the character of subsequent lymphopoiesis in scattered lymphoid organs. However, the overall rates of lymphopoiesis (through DNA synthesis) may be affected by events which trans-

pire in the thymus (as mentioned in the preceding paragraph).

Finally, the following considerations may be of particular immunologic as well as trophic significance.

1. In multiple lymphoid organs, the direct reutilization of large quantities of DNA from circulating lymphocytes along with large quantities of simpler circulating substances from their rich arterial circulation will supply the genetic information and substrate necessary to the continuous neoformation of large numbers of short-lived lymphocytes having immunologic, genetic, and other characteristics similar to circulating lymphocytes. It will also supply the genetic information and substrate necessary for the continuous production of large quantities of plasma and plasma proteins having immunologic and other characteristics similar to their short-lived counterparts* which are produced while the short-lived lymphocytes are differentiating and growing in the lymphoid organs (see Chap. 9).

2. In the germinal centers of multiple lymphoid organs, the indirect reutilization of small quantities of DNA from circulating lymphocytes along with small quantities of simpler substances from a poor arterial circulation will allow for periodic changes in the character of the precursors of short-lived lymphocytes produced there. This depends on the nature of simpler circulating substances utilized in histiocytes (along with the lymphocytic DNA) and fed back from the histiocytes to the mesenchymal reticular cells which, in turn, differentiate into multiple cell types, including lymphocytes ultimately destined to circulate into another part of the same organ or onward into the systemic circulation. (Such reutilization of circulating lymphocyte DNA along with antigenic substrate in the histiocytes of the germinal centers of multiple lymphoid organs may well have a great deal to do with the quantity of immunologically competent cells and antibodies produced, as well as the rapidity with which they are produced in quantity, during the secondary immunologic reaction. This is opposed to the primary immunologic reaction dur-

---

* While it is not known at what rate each constituent of the plasma turns over, isotopic studies indicate that the plasma proteins are replaced in the healthy individual every 2 to 28 days, depending on the specific protein in question.[166,167]

ing which the lymphatic sinusoids and parasinusoidal reticulum of regional lymphoid organs are primarily involved (see Chap. 18).

3. Whereas the former (direct) type of reutilization of lymphocyte DNA, along with simpler substances, makes allowance for stability of character in the relatively large quantities of lymphocytes and plasma produced to be reutilized in other lymphoid or nonlymphoid tissues, the latter (indirect) type of reutilization will allow for modification in the character of lymphocytes and plasma produced in many different lymphoid organs under changing physiologic or substrate situations, so that aliquots of lymphocytes and plasma may be utilized in other lymphoid and nonlymphoid tissues for more than one purpose (see Chap. 18). This may explain why a significant proportion of the plasma proteins or 1 to 2 percent of the circulating small lymphocytes [272] at any given time, will be found to be capable of prompt and specific reaction [272] toward any one of 10,000 to 20,000 potential antigens, whereas the remaining plasma proteins and lymphocytes not actually committed to this purpose at the given time remain capable of reacting to many other antigens while carrying on other feeding functions.

f. *The Germinal Centers and the Secondary Lymph Follicles*

Germinal centers and secondary lymph follicles are lacking in coelenterates and vertebrates which breathe by gills and lacking in the lymphoid tissues of air-breathing vertebrates prior to birth.[125,128,168] With birth and the changeover from oxygenation via the gills or the placenta to oxygenation via the lungs, the changeover from vitelline (yolk sac and placental) nutrition to oral feeding, and the commencement of age involution in the thymus, the germinal centers commence to appear in the intestinal lymphoid tissue, spleen, and lymph nodes.[6,125] At the same time, the Hassall's corpuscles commence to develop, more or less simultaneously, in the thymus.[125,164] (If the thymus is removed at the time of birth or shortly thereafter, the development of germinal centers is greatly retarded.[24]) Comparing different species of vertebrates, the degree of development of germinal centers increases with increasing development of the arterial system, an increasing arteriovenous oxygen difference, and an increasing basal metabolic rate [74,128] (or, simply, with the amount of oxygen normally assimilated per unit of time per unit of mass under basal conditions).

In normal neonatal mammals, the germinal centers appear first in the Peyer's patches of the small intestinal lymphoid tissue [168] (probably when the latter begins to undergo hypertrophy and cellular hyperplasia in conjunction with the absorption of ingested food). Subsequently, they develop in the spleen and lymph nodes [23,29,74,147,168] but normally do not develop in the thymus [2,164] or in the periarteriolar lymphoid tissue of the marrow. [148] The degree of germinal center development in the organs mentioned is generally maximal at the time of puberty when the thymus achieves greatest absolute weight (see Introduction) and the basal metabolic rate reaches its peak, compared with the rate during childhood or adult life. [128]

In lymph organs in which germinal centers develop, they do so alongside afferent muscular arterioles where the arterioles leave fibrous septa to enter the lymphoid tissue proper. Each usually receives a tiny capillary branch from the afferent arteriole as it commences to ramify into arcuate branches supplying the lymphocytes in the follicles and before it continues into the straight branch which carries on through the secondary and primary follicles into the medullary reticulum (as described earlier). As already mentioned, the germinal center capillary, when found, appears to be lined in its midportion by cells which resemble sinusoidal endothelium. The latter components of the capillary, in turn, are surrounded by heterogenous, syncytially arranged mesenchymal cells similar to those surrounding the venous sinusoids of the splenic red pulp. With respect to injected acid colloidal dyes, injected foreign proteins, spontaneous and experimentally induced infections, and stimuli which result in myeloid metaplasia, the reactions of the cells lining and surrounding the midportion of the germinal center capillary in those lymphoid organs which contain germinal centers are similar to the reactions of the sinusoidal endothelium and surrounding mesenchymal elements in the splenic red pulp.[37,38,169] One may therefore regard the midportion of the germinal center capillary and the surrounding mesenchymal elements as active mesenchyme similar to that in the splenic red pulp.[38] But it is active mesenchyme located in Peyer's patches, the spleen, and lymph nodes very close to the points of entrance of afferent arterioles into the lymphoid tissue proper in these various organs. In this sentinel position, this active mesenchyme in the germinal centers differs from that in the splenic red pulp in that all incoming substrate comes almost directly from systemic arterial blood. All its cellular progeny and cellular products must either spin off into the immediately surrounding lymphoid tissue population or flow onward into the medullary reticulum.

It should be added, for orientational purposes, that the active mesenchyme in the splenic red pulp may receive substrate not only directly from thoroughfare arteries [37,131] but also indirectly from germinal centers, the secondary and primary follicles, and the medullary reticulum, all of which ultimately drain their cells and cellular products via open channels in the reticulum toward the sinusoids.[37,131] Moreover, in the splenic red pulp, the cellular progeny and cellular products of the local active mesenchyme must spin off either into adjacent cells or into the portal venous sinusoids draining into the liver.[37] Thus the orientation of the active mesenchyme in the splenic red pulp differs from that of the germinal centers in general.

In order to understand the role of the germinal centers in relation to lymphopoiesis in the spleen, nodes, and Peyer's patches; and why [3]HT-labeling patterns differ in different types of lymph follicles, it is necessary to consider that significant numbers of circulating lymphocytes (particularly those formed in the intestinal lymphoid tissue) do not become labeled. Consider the fact that the cell reactions in the germinal centers are phasic [8,96,170] and that arterial blood flow in the follicles is phasic also.[131,155,156] The active mesenchyme of the germinal centers may be profoundly affected by the cell and protein content of the blood which enters at any given moment via the relatively small germinal center capillary. But the lymphocytes growing in the surrounding reticulum may be affected not only by what is going on in the germinal center but also by the phasic manner in which arterial blood flows through the arcuate channels over periods of time. With ebb-and-flow cycles which may vary from minute to minute or hour to hour and yet involve relatively large volumes (as observed directly by MacKenzie [131]), and which may evolute and involute over a period of a few days (as observed by Jaeger [155] and Maximow [156]), it is possible that events which transpire in the germinal centers may seem out of phase with events which transpire in the lymphocytes surrounding these centers (see Fig. 45).

As pointed out by Conway,[170] the reticulum (active mesenchyme) of germinal centers passes through a phase during which histiocytic digestion of nuclei and other debris, and one wherein neoformation of large and giant lymphocytes, appears to predominate. During the first, or reaction, phase, usually the germinal center will be surrounded by a mantle zone of densely packed small lymphocytes which label poorly with ^{3}HT.[55,98] During the second, or proliferative, phase, the germinal centers will be surrounded by large and medium-sized lymphocytes which seem to radiate from the germinal centers and seem to emanate from the large lymphocytes in the germinal centers,[8,96,147,170] all of which seem to label quite heavily.[55,98] Surrounding the germinal centers in the proliferative phase and the large and medium-sized lymphocytes which grow from there outward, the mantle zone of small, densely packed, poorly labeled lymphocytes may be displaced outward, thus giving rise to layered nodules called tertiary nodules by Ehrich.[96,171] As pointed out by Ehrich [96,171] and more recently by Fleidner *et al.*,[55] by comparing the lymphoid nodules in different portions of the cortex of a given lymphoid organ, all three types of nodules—primary, secondary, and tertiary—may be found simultaneously.

On the basis of disparity in phase times, one may readily explain why the compressed small lymphocytes in the mantle zones surrounding the germinal centers in reaction phase, as they appear in many secondary lymph nodules and surrounding the reactive and proliferative germinal centers of tertiary nodules, appear to bear no geneological relationship to the germinal centers which they surround. For if the phase of reaction in the germinal centers is shorter than the phase of lymphocyte growth in conjunction with active arterial flow through the arcuate channels, there will always be evidence of reaction centers springing up to displace the small lymphocytes which have been generated previously from adjacent primary, secondary, or tertiary nodules.

In other words, new reaction centers do not necessarily generate the small lymphocytes in the surrounding mantle zones but primarily push aside small lymphocytes generated previously from other sources. Thus, if one studies the problem in terms of ³HT labeling, he will find an obvious disparity in the grain counts in giant lymphocytes (germinoblasts) and large lymphocytes forming in the germinal centers of the reaction type, as compared with the grain counts in the small, compressed lymphocytes surrounding these centers, whereas evidence of such disparity will be lacking in the adjacent primary follicles.

Estimates of actual reaction phase time in germinal centers of secondary lymph follicles vs. the total time it takes for germinal centers to react, become transformed into proliferative centers of tertiary nodules, and ultimately give rise to circulating small lymphocytes can be made by comparing the time it takes for peak labeling to occur in the large lymphocytes of the germinal centers with the total time it takes for immunologic reactions primarily involving the germinal centers to occur. Peak labeling in the giant and large lymphocytes (DNA synthesis time) of the germinal centers is observed to take place at about five hours with ³HT,[55] whereas it takes approximately two to three days for the centers to undergo the whole series of reactions which culminate in the delivery of significant numbers of immunologically competent small lymphocytes to the circulation after one or more previous exposures to antigens emanating from foreign cells (see Chap. 18) . Therefore, it can be estimated that actual reaction time in the germinal centers is five hours, whereas total reaction-proliferation-release time is on the order of two to three days.

Noting, however, that ³HT probably diffuses more slowly than

$^{32}PO_4$ and that peak labeling with each type of isotope-labeled DNA precursor differs by a factor of approximately 5, one may assume further that it takes about 1 hour for the reaction phase in the germinal centers to take place, whereas it takes 48 to 72 hours for large numbers of immunologically competent lymphocytes to start appearing in the circulating blood during the secondary immunologic response. One should note, then, that such figures compare favorably with Leblond's [121] and Everett's [98,117] estimates on how long it takes reticular cells to transform into lymphocytes and the estimates of median total life span of lymphocytes as calculated by Yoffey.[115] Subtracting the one-hour reaction-phase time from the total time it takes the secondary immunologic response to appear, one is left with a 47- to 71-hour lymphocyte differentiation and proliferation time in the reticulum surrounding the germinal centers where the growing, dividing medium-sized and small lymphocytes are well supplied with arterial blood via the arcuate arterioles. Therefore, one may calculate that the time from evolution to involution as described by Jaeger,[155] and the arterial flow phase in average secondary germinal centers may be on the order of two to three days.

In support of these considerations are the observations of Millikin [287-289] who, like Jaeger and Maximow, studied the germinal centers in the third dimension by serial sections. Millikin found the following (see Figs. 46–52).

1. Germinal centers appear to expand rapidly, as evidenced by their rapid growth during the course of fulminating infections and by the compressed appearance of stroma and small lymphocytes in mantle zones surrounding them.

2. The centers grow as bipolar spheroids which, if bisected in a plane perpendicular to the polar axis, will yield a dark-staining hemispheroid whose pole is always adjacent to the afferent arterial supply of the germinal center, and a pale-staining hemispheroid whose pole is always oriented away from the afferent arterial supply toward mucosal surfaces (in the case of the oropharyngeal, bronchial, and intestinal lymphoid tissue) or toward the afferent lymph sinuses (in the case of the nodes).

3. Both the dark- and pale-staining hemispheroids normally contain relatively large numbers of pyknotic nuclear fragments, ostensibly the remains of small lymphocytes. Millikin interpreted this finding to indicate that the germinal centers normally reutilize nuclear material, and the information contained, from small lymphocytes.

4. The mantle zone of small lymphocytes appears thinner and more compressed at the pole of the juxtaarteriolar hemispheroid than at the abarteriolar pole of germinal centers. This finding can be interpreted to indicate that growth and expansion of germinal center cells is most rapid toward their arterial blood supply (from which these cells are obliged to receive the substrate necessary for growth).

5. Surrounding the mantle zone which consists of tightly packed, small lymphocytes, the perifollicular zone, made up of medium-sized lymphocytes, forms a continuum with the periarteriolar (medium-sized) lymphocyte sheath which surrounds and follows the course of the arterioles in the spleen and other organized lymphoid tissues. At the arteriolar poles of germinal centers where mantle zones are thinnest and often disrupted, a continuum seems apparent between the larger and medium-sized lymphocytes of the germinal center and the medium-sized lymphocytes to be found in the perifollicular zone and periarteriolar lymphocyte sheath. These findings can be interpreted to indicate that the germinal centers indeed give rise to the lymphocytes which lie between and surround them but do so primarily at their arterial poles where the supply of substrate is most plentiful.

At the abarterial poles where the blood supply is less plentiful, the mantle zones will consist, then, of lymphocytes which were differentiated from other germinal centers or primary lymph follicles at an earlier date but are compressed by the inordinately rapid growth of new germinal centers (see Figs. 46–51).

6. The dark-staining hemispheroid in well-developed germinal centers contains relatively great numbers of large, basophilic (pyroninophilic), mitotically active cells resembling large lymphocytes. Hence, there is a dark, relatively basophilic staining

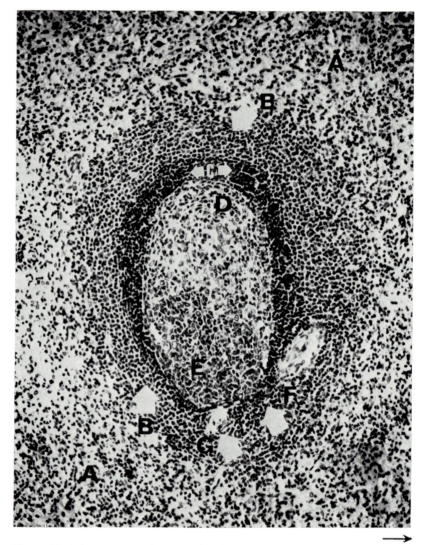

Figure 46. A human secondary lymph follicle sectioned precisely in polar axis × 240. A, Medulla consisting largely of reticular connective tissue (reticulum) and phagocytic mononuclear cells surrounding sinusoids, venous (in the case of the spleen) or lymphatic (in the case of the nodes). B. Perifollicular envelope consisting mostly of medium-sized lymphocytes embedded in an attenuated reticular matrix. C. Mantle zone consisting of compressed, small cytoplasm-poor lymphocytes embedded in a very compressed, attenuated reticular matrix. D. Pale pole of germinal center consisting largely of reticu-

quality in the juxtaarteriolar hemispheroid. The abarteriolar pale-staining hemispheroid is composed principally of reticular cells and histiocytes whose nuclei have less affinity for basic dyes and whose cytoplasm is eosinophilic or amphophilic. (This indicates a lower concentration of reactive acid phosphate groups and a relatively low concentration of nuclear DNA and cytoplasmic RNA in comparison with the dark (basophilic) staining cells in the juxtaarteriolar hemispheroid.) Any section cut at an angle to the polar axis will yield a distorted estimate of the relative numbers of dark-staining and pale-staining cells, depending on which hemispheroid occupies the bulk of the section (see Fig. 52). If the cut is predominantly through the juxtaarteriolar hemispheroid, relatively great numbers of large basophilic cells will be transected (and the sectioned cells may be expected to show a relatively high rate of incorporation of nucleic acid precursors, such as ^{3}HT or ^{32}PO$_4$). If the cut is predominently through the abarteriolar hemispheroid, mostly pale cells with a relatively low order of mitotic activity will be transected (and the sectioned cells may be expected to show a relatively low order of labeled mucleic acid precursors, as compared with cuts through the former).

Thus in sections which are cut at random with respect to their polar axes, different germinal centers sectioned may show seemingly different cell populations (and varying uptake of labeled DNA precursors), particularly in the spleen where orientation toward mucosal surfaces or afferent lymph sinuses is lacking and

lar cells and histiocytes. E. Dark pole of germinal center consisting mainly of large deeply basophilic lymphocytes and reticular cells. F. Periarteriolar lymphoid tissue sheath consisting principally of medium-sized and small lymphocytes embedded in the reticular stroma surrounding the arterioles. G. Afferent arteriole of the germinal center.

Note the relatively great thickness of the mantle zone, or "cap" surrounding the pale pole of the germinal center, as compared with the thickness of the mantle zone surrounding the dark, juxtaarteriolar pole. Note also in this and ensuing Figures 47 to 51 how the mantle zone seems to disappear near the afferent arteriole, so that cells of the dark pole of the germinal center appear to become confluent with the medium-sized and smaller lymphocytes in the pariarteriolar lymphoid tissue sheath. From Millikin, P. D.[289]

react and produce the precursors of lymphocytes which subsequently can be characterized by immunologic methods. As already mentioned earlier, important forms of substrate in directing the character of lymphocytes to be produced may be endogenous proteins and DNA from circulating lympocytes, as well as exogenous free extracellular proteins. Moreover, all of the latter are normally carried in via the small germinal center capillaries, not just in one lymphoid organ, but almost simultaneously in many (owing to mixing during circulation).

Second, it requires relatively large quantities of additional substrate, as well as a longer period of time, for the characterized or "immunologically committed" lymphocyte precursors to consummate growth and mitotic division into the relatively large, morphologically homogeneous lymphocyte population which grows to surround the arterioles and lie between the germinal centers. Important forms of substrate are water, oxygen, glucose, salts, amino acids, fats, and free DNA precursors, regardless of their labeling with isotopes of given elements. Moreover, all must be supplied in relatively large quantity via the arterioles which the lymphocytes grow to surround and which the arterioles correspondingly increase their flow to supply (see Fig. 45) not just in one lymphoid organ but in many.

A third consideration is that over extended periods of time in multiple lymphoid organs, individual germinal centers and zones of surrounding lymphocytes grow and disappear, to be replaced by others. Throughout these organs, the rates of germinal center and secondary follicle growth appear accelerated by many factors, including the presence of infection, a relatively high tissue oxygen tension, an adequate supply of substrate from ingested food, and the presence of thymic entodermal hormone which accelerates DNA synthesis in the lymphocytes. The rate of their disappearance, individually and collectively, appears accelerated by multiple factors, including anoxia, starvation, stress, and the presence of adrenal glucocorticoids which induce lymphocytolysis, especially in the mantle zones.

As already mentioned, since they are lacking in veins and lymphatics, the germinal and mantle zones not only receive the substrate necessary for growth from systemic arteries but also must discharge their cells and lytic products into the arteries or into the environs. Therefore, their cells and their cellular products must circulate first through the paracortical and medullary portions of the mother lymphoid organ or organs before gaining access to the general circulation via veins or efferent lymphatics.

As already mentioned also, some of the cells or their products may be utilized for lymphopoiesis in the paracortical and medullary portions of mother lymphoid organs. Those which pass through unutilized, then, must be collected via lymphatics and veins to circulate back to the mother lymphoid organ, to other lymphoid organs, to the thymus, and to remaining organs in the body. In each of these areas, the reutilization of the cells or their free extracellular products must have appreciable consequences.

In other lymphoid organs, as well as in the mother lymphoid organ, the reutilization of DNA and possibly other substances from circulating lymphocytes which have originated from one or more secondary lymph follicles will allow for increased lymphopoiesis in certain lymphoid organs at the expense of others. Moreover, as already mentioned, such reutilization will allow for the accelerated dissemination of genetic material from one to all and all to one, more or less simulaneously. Thus a relatively rich arterial supply in each lymphoid organ assures opportunity for quantitatively important reutilization (such as has been shown to occur by the isotope data cited earlier). As a consequence of reutilization, each of the lymphoid organs containing germinal centers may give rise to great numbers of additional lymphocytes carrying similar old, and additional new, genetic codes, without having to completely process a new antigen locally and without having to increase significantly the ambient rate of small lymphocyte production.

In the thymus, the rate of feedback and consequent reutilization of DNA (and possibly other substances) from circulating lymphocytes gaining random access to Hassall's corpuscles (as suggested in sect. 1) may reduce the rate of hormone production by the epithelial reticular cells and thus reduce the overall rate of germinal center growth and small lymphocyte production throughout the lymphoid organs. Such feedback regulation of thymic hormonal output has been proven experimentally by Nagaya *et al.*,[172] who showed that the rate of DNA synthesis in thymocytes is accelerated by circulating lymphocytopenia and decelerated by circulating lymphocytosis. That the Hassall's corpuscles are critically involved in this feedback mechanism is suggested not only by the microscopic observations outlined above but also by the fact that their number increases while thymic hormonal output appears to decrease with age.[16]

In remaining organs, the consequences of reutilization will be considered at length later.

In summary, then, one may envision the germinal centers and the secondary lymph follicles within lymphoid organs as specialized organoids whose development parallels phylogenetic evolution, evolution of the arterial system, evolution of an increasing arteriovenous oxygen difference, and increasing development of the thymus; as organoids whose substrate supply is entirely via systemic arteries; and as organoids whose differentiated products drain via open arterial channels into the paracortical and medullary reticulum of lymphoid organs. Under normal conditions when the individual is feeding and breathing normally, one of their important functions would appear to be to consume free extracellular substrate and substrate from circulating cells as "reaction centers" which, in turn, germinate large numbers of small lymphocytes to carry substrate and appropriate genetic information to other lymphoid and nonlymphoid organs via the circulatory system, a process accelerated by the secretion of a hormone from the entodermal cells of the thymus. Under abnormal conditions, when the individual is starving, anoxic, or under severe stress, one of their important functions would appear to be to release their substance through rapid cytolysis, especially in the mantle zones, a process accelerated by secretion of adrenal glucocorticoids. Finally, because the germinal centers (not just in one, but in many lymphoid organs) are oriented toward and dependent primarily on their afferent arterioles for the substrate essential to growth and differentiation, all may be envisioned as centers where new information brought in by circulating plasma and cells is assimilated with old information carried by circulating plasma and cells, to the end that new generations of lymphocytes may be kept properly informed to carry on various tasks, whether they be purely trophic or purely immunologic (see Chap. 18). Thus, like universities, they may be looked upon as centers of learning, well designed to blend information which is new with information which is old or classic, so that maximal graduates may proceed, optimally prepared to deal with the world in which they live.

g. Summary and Conclusions

The introduction into the body of compounds containing radioactive isotopes of naturally occurring elements in chemically identical, biologically active compounds has yielded valuable information in the study of cellular kinetics, particularly in lymphocytes which incorporate isotope-labeled DNA precursors at a relatively rapid rate in comparison with remaining body cells. It has been found that many lymphocytes in organized lymphoid tissues and circulating blood incorporate isotope-labeled DNA precursors, such as radioactive phosphate ($^{32}PO_4$) and tritiated thymidine (^3HT), at a very rapid rate, whereas some lymphocytes in the lymphoid organs and blood do not. Therefore, many have assumed (and it is currently considered proven) that the body contains lymphocytes of long, as well as short, biologic life, an assumption compatible with the stem cell concept of small lymphocyte function and an assumption upon which many of the currently popular conclusions outlined above are based.

Through analysis of data on cellular, thoracic duct lymph, and lymphoid organ changes following the absorption of food, it is shown that the aforementioned assumption is incorrect. For during the days, weeks, or months which transpire during experiments involving the injection and autoradiographic tracing of isotope-labeled DNA precursors, the experimental animal, in order to survive and grow, must continue to absorb similar unlabeled DNA precursors via the gastrointestinal tract, particularly

and a hormone which accelerates DNA synthesis in lymphocytes generally.

7. In the bone marrow, as compared with cells of the granulocytic, erythroid, or thrombocytic series, lymphoid cells incorporate relatively large quantities of the label from labeled, transfused heterologous lymphocytes.[102] This finding, together with the finding that labeled as well as unlabeled thoracic duct lymphocytes and thymic lymphocytes appear relatively incapable of repopulating the bone marrow of heavily irradiated animals,[23] has lent little evidence to suggest that the small lymphocyte by itself functions as a stem cell for granulocytes, erythrocytes, or thrombocytes (see B, above).

8. Finally, it is noteworthy that there is no clear-cut data to indicate at what rate the labeled cells or their label disappear from the lymphoid and myeloid organs, appear within non-hematopoietic tissues, appear as free precursors or precursors bound to free extracellular proteins, and appear within the urine and feces, as measured for extended periods of time (e.g. 100–300 days).

The data obtained by injecting labeled lymphocytes, although supplementary to the data obtained by direct *in vivo* labeling with DNA precursors, have not differentiated clearly whether the small circulating lymphocyte is a stem cell or a trephocyte. The fact that injected isotope-labeled lymphocytes from selected sources appear to "home" to relatively specific sites, primarily in the lymphoid organs and in the liver points to the stem cell concept.[23,72,177,178] Homing to the sinusoids of the spleen and liver, however, may indicate that the bulk of injected cells, particularly from the thymus (where cells are extremely radiosensitive and stress lymphocytolysis is very prone to take place) or cells labeled *in vitro* (where damage owing to labeling and handling may be expected) are nonviable and therefore handled *in vivo* like other foreign proteins or large molecules injected intravenously.[38] Homing to medullary (paracortical) reticulum of the nodes and spleen may be interpreted in two ways. First, relatively large numbers of viable cells, particularly from the thoracic duct (where minimal manipulation is required to obtain motile, viable, almost pure suspensions of lymphocytes), take up residence in the medullary (paracortical) reticulum where they commence to differentiate into plasmacytes and lymphocytes which, in turn, proliferate. Second, owing to a relatively rich arterial circulation, a relatively large proportion of the labeled DNA from viable injected lymphocytes is reutilized in the medullary (paracortical) reticulum in a manner similar to that from labeled endogenous circulating lymphocytes (see E, above).

Supplementing the second interpretation other items in favor of the trephocytic or trophic concept of small lymphocyte function are as follows.

1. In other tissues besides lymphoid tissue where the cellular growth rate is known to be relatively rapid (e.g. in normal crypt epithelium of the small intestine,[94] in regenerating hepatic polygonal cells,[43,44] in fibroblasts of healing wounds,[42] and in sarcomas (ascites tumors) of mice [179]), the isotope label from injected labeled lymphocytes is incorporated at a relatively rapid rate also. Such incorporation of label from the injected lymphocytes can be interpreted to indicate that the donor lymphocytes transform into intestinal crypt epithelium, hepatic polygonal cells, fibroblasts, or sarcoma cells in the host—or that they have donated their DNA to the latter. While there is some evidence to indicate that lymphocytes may be transformed into fibroblasts,[22] there is little evidence that they are transformed directly into intestinal crypt epithelium, hepatic polygonal cells, or mouse sarcomas (ascites tumors). Therefore, it seems most likely that they donate their DNA, or at least their labeled precursors ($^{32}PO_4$ or ^3HT), to other types of cells whose rate of growth happens to be relatively rapid at the time of injection.

2. The virtual disappearance of injected isotope-labeled lymphocytes [180,181] or acridine-labeled lymphocytes [174] from the blood and lymph of the recipient within 30 to 90 minutes confirms Yoffey's earlier calculations [115] that the intravascular life span of small lymphocytes is normally on the order of one to two hours in healthy small animals. Moreover, such a rapid rate of disappearance detracts from the theory that there is normally a quantitatively important recirculation of small lymphocytes from

blood to lymph via the nodes and mitigates against a prolonged small-lymphocyte life span, if evidence for recirculation is to be considered evidence for prolonged total life span.

3. In lethally irradiated animals in which there is an acute need for new lymphoid and myeloid cells, the failure of injected labeled lymphocytes to produce effective repopulation of the blood-forming organs mitigates directly against the stem cell hypothesis.

4. In hematologically normal animals (and humans) wherein there is no obvious need for extraneous lymphoid cells, myeloid cells, or other formed elements, both isotope-labeled [180,181] and karyotype-labeled [73] donor lymphocytes disappear from the circulation within one to two hours. However, karyotype-labeled lymphocytes reappear in the circulation in numbers three to seven times the number injected within relatively few hours.[73] Meanwhile, isotope-labeled cells (or their labels) fail to reappear in significant quantity in the circulating blood, and are found in various kinds of cells in the liver reticulum, bone marrow, spleen, nodes, connective tissues, and short-lived epithelia (as outlined previously). These data may be explained on the following bases.

First, even though he has no need for them, injected karyotype-labeled lymphocytes colonize, proliferate in, and disseminate from hemopoietic organs of the host and give rise to so many lymphocytes (and, possibly, other types of cells) carrying the donor karyotype that the isotope label becomes too dilute to measure.

Second, the injected karyotype-labeled lymphocytes, as they colonize, proliferate, and disseminate under the same conditions, replicate similar genetic characteristics within their lymphocytic progeny, but dissociate the isotope label from their DNA into many kinds of lymphoid and nonlymphoid cells.

Third, the DNA from injected karyotype-labeled lymphocytes is reutilized quantitatively, and the genetic characteristic temporarily expressed in rapidly growing host lymphocytes and, possibly, in other types of cells (see below). Meanwhile, the quantities of isotope-labeled DNA injected become so heavily diluted by naturally acquired DNA precursors that labeled DNA becomes too dilute and disseminate to measure by the methods employed currently.

In the light of foregoing data, analysis will reveal the third possibility to be most likely.

G. SMALL-LYMPHOCYTE TO MACROPHAGE TRANSFORMATION

Morphologic study of cells obtained by touching or smearing experimentally produced inflammatory exudates onto slides, and examining them at various time intervals during the course of the inflammatory reaction by standard hematologic techniques are interpreted to indicate that small lymphocytes which emmigrate from the blood into the interstices are capable of undergoing direct transformation into macrophages,[182] just as some appear to do in tissue culture.[28,183] It has been disputed, however, whether such findings prove the lymphocytic origin of macrophages under normal, as well as under all abnormal, situations [72] or that they supply a clinching proof of the stem cell theory.[96] Many researchers consider the macrophages to be of mesenchymal or histogenous origin from reticular (adventitial) cells in the connective tissues.[28-39] Morphologic studies on exudate cells containing isotope label, after previous injection of [3]HT, are interpreted to indicate that macrophages are transformed from monocytes which have their origin in the bone marrow [72] (where a relatively high and early rate of labeling of medium-sized mononuclear cells takes place after intravenous injection of [3]HT- see Fig. 38). Origin of the macrophages from more than one of the aforementioned sources is currently considered to be most likely.[72]

It is significant from a morphologic point of view that during the early stages of cytolysis, lymphocytes (like many other cells) may undergo swelling owing to the cellular imbibition of water (potocytosis).[39] As a result of this swelling, they may take on the appearance of macrophages having abundant, foamy cytoplasm and relatively large leptochromatic (as opposed to small pachychromatic) nuclei. If some are labeled by previous injection of [3]HT (regardless of the organ in which they are labeled) and they disintegrate, their label will become available for reutilization

cytes growing in PHA tissue-culture systems results in their production of specific agglutinins toward the given antigen.[187]

In vivo after injection of purified extracts of lymphocytes obtained from sensitized donor, a lag period of four to six hours ensues when no lymphocytes demonstrating immunologic reactivity or immunologic memory for the antigen can be recovered from the blood of the nonsensitized recipient.[187] After 18 to 24 hours, large numbers can be recovered consistently.[187] It will be noted, then, that the lag period and the rate of appearance of such sensitized lymphocytes (possessing immunologic memory) in the circulating blood of the recipient corresponds very closely to the lag period and rate of appearance of lymphocytes of foreign karyotype in the blood after their injection into a non-irradiated human recipient (see B, above). The former type of injection would appear to differ from the latter primarily in the period of time that altered lymphocytes are demonstrable in the blood. Whereas the purified lymphocyte extracts contain little protein and may imprint an immunologic memory code into the DNA of the recipient's lymphocytes demonstrable for one to two years, the whole lymphocytes of foreign karyotype contain proteins and disappear from the circulating blood of the recipient in seven to ten days (unless the individual has been immunologically paralyzed by neonatal thymectomy, radiation, or other immunosuppressive measures).

These findings indicate that it is not necessarily whole-donor lymphocytes which take up residence, proliferate, and migrate in the recipient but, more likely, small molecules, presumably from small-lymphocyte DNA, which induce morphologic or functional alterations in proliferating lymphocytes of the recipient. This conclusion is supported not only by the data outlined earlier but also by very recent observations that purified DNA from organs of pigmented mice, when passed through mesenchymal cells of albino mice, can induce pigmentation in healthy albinos of the same species.[193] Thus, it would appear that the genetic code of donor DNA fragments can be expressed in mammalian cells in a manner analogous to that which occurs in bacteria. Therefore, it would appear that small lymphocytes do not function as stem cells in some of these situations, but as donors of information via their DNA (or its fragments) and as donors of information which can be expressed in recipient cells.

Chapter 17

REDUCTIO AD ABSURDUM
A. THE LYMPHOCYTE DISPOSITION PROBLEM—
A GAME OF NUMBERS

TO THOSE SUCH as Yoffey,[74-76,85,101-102,115,128] who have long studied the mass and distribution of lymphocytes in the body as well as the lymphokinetic data recently obtained through the use of isotopes, the disposition of lymphocytes poses a fascinating problem, particularly if their lifespan is considered to be finite— whether it be 2 to 4 days in the lymphoid organs and 1 to 2 hours in the circulating blood, or 90 to 300 days total with continual recirculation between blood and lymph. Although it seems clear to the microscopist that many small lymphocytes disintegrate in lymphoid organs, either as isolated cells or within macrophages,[140,141] it seems clear also that many large and medium-sized lymphocytes are dividing and showing progressive evidence of differentiation in the same areas at the same time.[140,141] As the biologic purpose of simultaneous degeneration and regeneration in the organized lymphoid tissues is not entirely obvious at first glance, many researchers have looked toward other areas where small lymphocyte disposition may be demonstrable. Some have considered that large numbers may be excreted into the lumen of the intestine, but others have shown that although such excretion takes place, the numbers appear negligible as compared with the total produced. Showing that the number of marrow lymphocytes varies inversely with the erythropoietic (reticulocyte) response to anoxia, Yoffey has continually advocated that relatively large numbers of lymphocytes serve as precursors for erythrocytes. Lacking definitive proof that lymphocytes undergo heteroplastic differentiation into erythroblasts and finding by isotope-labeling techniques that the marrow serves as a center of active lymphocytopoiesis, he continues to pursue the lymphocyte disposition problem, stating: "They just seem to disappear into the blue." [194] Although vague, such a statement seems prophetic to those accustomed to studying formed elements and disintegrating lymphocytes in Romanowsky-stained smears of bone marrow aspirate and sections stained by other methods. Under the eyes of the microscopist, out of the blue-staining nuclear material, radiates the information, and out of the blue-staining plasma and ground substance are imbibed the substrate from which the differentiation and growth of red-staining cells, leucocytes, and megakaryocytes in the marrow are consummated.

As already mentioned and discussed (Chap. 16, G) Rebuck *et al.*[182] have presented controversial evidence indicating that small lymphocytes differentiate into macrophages during inflammation. The consideration that many lymphocytes ultimately differentiate into plasmacytes or recirculate for prolonged periods of time, as proposed by Gowans,[72] remains popular currently and is discussed in several portions of the text (Chaps. 9, 11, and 16, C). Still others have looked toward rapidly growing epithelia and connective tissues as the ultimate graveyard of many circulating lymphocytes, as shown in the photomicrographs in Section 1 of this text and which will be discussed subsequently in more detail.

The fact remains that if significant numbers of lymphocytes are cells which grow rapidly and are of short life span, as is indicated by the isotope data as well as other forms of data summarized, disposition remains a serious problem. If they are cells of long as well as short biologic life, as is indicated by current interpretations of the isotope and karyotype data, one must provide a satisfactory explanation for the disposition of both the short-lived and the long-lived lymphocytes. In terms of substance donation to an almost unlimited number and variety of cells, one may explain the disposition of an almost unlimited number of small lymphocytes, whether they be long-lived or short-lived. The question arises, then, of whether one can explain the disposition of almost unlimited numbers of short-lived as well as long-lived lymphocytes by their differentiation into a limited variety of closely related cells whose numbers in the body relative to the number of small lymphocytes are normally small.

remaining tissues. As the spleen proceeds to become the largest single lymphoid organ in the body, while the thymus is undergoing its characteristic pattern of shrinkage with age, it may be envisoned as a progressively important storage depot of proteins and nucleic acids, as well as an organ dynamically concerned with humoral immunity and the turnover of circulating blood constituents, as outlined in Section 1. Its surgical removal, interestingly enough, results only in transient hypoproteinemia and a slightly increased incidence of serious infection in children, perhaps owing to the fact that it normally constitutes one sixth to one fourth of the total lymphoid tissue mass and to the fact that splenectomy may be followed by compensatory hyperplasia of lymphoid elements surrounding the arterioles in the portal triads of the liver and surrounding the arterioles in the marrow.

d. Lymph Nodes

Having been primed similarly by contributions from the thymus, and proceeding to receive substrate circulated from the intestinal lymphoid tissue, the liver, and the spleen, the lymph nodes grow to reutilize, store, and release substance in the form of lymph, doing so in quantities which may seem relatively small in comparison with the potential in the thymus, intestinal lymphoid tissue, and spleen.[132,133] However, in addition, they receive substrate emanating from the peripheral tissues and carried in via their afferent lymphatics. The immunologic as well as nutritive significance of reutilization of the substrate from the periphery and from the systemic circulation will be discussed subsequently.

e. Lymphoid Tissue of the Bone Marrow

Primed similarly by circulating donations from the thymus and receiving additional substrate circulated from the intestinal lymphoid tissue, the liver (see Sect. 3), the spleen, and the efferent lymphatics of the nodes, the periarteriolar lymphoid tissue of the marrow grows to constitute approximately ten percent of the marrow cell population (e.g. 100 gm of lymphoid tissue) in the healthy, well-nourished, nonanoxic human adult. (In healthy children and small laboratory animals such as rats and mice, the percentage of lymphoid cells in the marrow may approach thirty percent). As shown by the isotope data cited earlier, this segment of the lymphoid tissue mass appears to incorporate labeled DNA precursors and therefore grow rapidly in comparison with remaining lymphoid organs (see Fig. 38). Morphologically, this segment consists of relatively large numbers of medium-sized or "transitional" lymphocytes [85] which appear to shed cytoplasm in an active manner (see Section 1). Therefore, as already mentioned, one may suspect that one of its important functions is to produce plasma which helps flush nonmotile formed elements such as erythrocytes and platelets into the venous sinusoids of the marrow so that the latter may commence circulation. As lymphatics are lacking in the marrow, that which remains of the marrow lymphoid cell population after shedding cytoplasm must migrate through the marrow reticulum to gain access to the venous sinusoids. In the myelopoietic tissue surrounding the sinusoids, the remaining protoplasm from the lymphoid cells (or its disintegration products) may be reutilized before passage into the sinusoids. Because many nuclear fragments in various stages of disintegration can be found in the reticulum and histiocytes of the marrow while developing erythrocytes and other myeloid cells appear to nurse on the cytoplasm of the latter, one may assume that some, if not many, of the cytoplasm-poor mononuclear cells, particularly the lymphocytes, donate their residual substance, mostly nuclear material, into a nucleic acid pool out of which other cells take sustenance.* This pool, consists of nuclear material obviously from other sources, such as circulating mononuclear and polymorphonuclear leucocytes; erythrocytes whose nuclei have been extruded, megakaryocytes whose nuclei do not circulate normally, and granulocytes which have commenced to disintegrate before circulating. It is

---

* Very recently, Heiniger et al. [290] have shown via isotope studies that rapidly growing cells in rat marrow, such as erythroblasts, megakaryocytes, and marrow lymphocytes, reutilize thymidine from "dead" cells. They have estimated that 40 to 60 percent of the thymidine in marrow blast cells is supplied from the DNA of "dead" cells. Moreover, they point to the presence of a "common thymidine pool" within the bone marrow.

region will all show a similar "secondary response." [23,60,96,210-213]
The latter is similar to the primary response outlined above in
that the same sequential cellular reactions take place but at a
greatly accelerated rate such that by the third day, small-lymphocyte production and the formation of germinal centers in the
follicles (see p. 185) is very obvious and somewhat obscures the
reaction of histiocytes and plasmacytes in the medullary reticulum
of the nodes.[23,60,96,210-213] The speed of the secondary response may
be due to the feedback into regional nodes of small quantities of
antibodies and small numbers of immunologically competent
small lymphocytes which have arisen as a result of previous exposure,[23,96,214,215] whereas the magnitude of the secondary response
may be owing to (random) feedback of similar entities into
the germinal centers of the secondary lymph follicles throughout
many scattered lymphoid organs (as outlined on pp. 203-205).

4. The ability to transfer delayed hypersensitivity reactions
from an immune donor to a nonimmune recipient of the same
general species by injection of small lymphocytes, heat-killed
lymphocytes, lyophilized lymphocytes, or lymphocytes implanted
in millipore diffusion chambers obtained from a donor who was
previously sensitized by the same antigen (see Chap. 16, H).

5. The finding *in vitro* that significant numbers of small lymphocytes from the circulating blood, when subsequently con-
fronted by a similar antigen, may resume RNA synthesis and
consummate the cytoplasmic synthesis of specific agglutinins toward this antigen. This occurs particularly when mitogens such
as PHA are added to the tissue culture medium (perhaps to dere-
press genetic characteristics which ordinarily would be repressed
by circulating plasma factors or circulating cells *in vivo* (see
Chap. 16, C and Lawrence [187]).

6. The prolonged persistence, continued production, and circulation of biologically short-lived agglutinins or immunoglobulins
(see Chap. 9) and biologically short-lived lymphocytes (see Chap.
16, E, 3) reactive to a specific antigen (and many others) for
many months and years after the regional node has shrunk to
normal size and its plasmacyte population has diminished to

mo   sys
ear   an
nor   ch
org   po
bac   for
tion
as   to
      wh
      cel
      loc
U   cell
isol cap
mal   suc
of t to
to   wei
so   cap
of s the
      and
1   the
      nod
      acce
      assu
      the
2.   to t
      part
      pro
      in t
      3.
      tioc
      cell
3.   may
      sup
      lym
      the
4.   Such
      inte
      beca

account for only 1 to 2 percent of total cells (see Chap. 9 and 10).

2. Sequential Cellular and Humoral Pathways Pursued by Antigenic Proteins

Taking a closer look at the pathways whereby antigenic proteins are processed, one may envision their tour through the lymphoid organs as follows.

1. Antigenic or not, free extracellular proteins emanating from cells and microbes can be cleared from the interstices to the regional nodes in two forms: (a) as unaltered free extracellular proteins which are carried to the regional nodes via peripheral lymphatics [38,74,128] or (b) as free extracellular proteins which have undergone phagocytosis within the interstices and are carried to the regional nodes via the peripheral lymphatics but carried in phagocytes or combined with the products of their disintegration.[38,74,128] (It is important to add here that peripheral lymph always flows through one or more regional nodes on its course from the periphery to the thoracic and cervical lymph ducts.[74,128])

2. On reaching the regional nodes, unaltered free extracellular proteins from the periphery and those which have suffered phagocytic digestion enter the nodal sinusoids where they may undergo phagocytosis and further digestion by histiocytes lining and surrounding the sinusoids [38] (and see p. 329). (It is important to add here that most free extracellular proteins which are recognizably antigenic are cleared from peripheral lymph and do not leave via efferent nodal lymph.[38,74,128])

3. After ingestion into histiocytes lining and surrounding the lymph sinusoids,[38,203] the free extracellular proteins may be digested and passed onward, either into the lymph sinusoids or into adjacent cells in which there lies further opportunity for digestion or addition of molecules. (See Fig. 1 where it will be noted that sequential cellular contiguity in lymphoid organs corresponds precisely to the sequential order of cellular reactions as a function of time described above, particularly during the primary immunologic response.)

phoid organs, to commence random migration) several events transpire almost simultaneously:

a. Small lymphocytes become the most numerous and prominent blood-borne cells in the damaged area.[13,201,202]

b. The microphages and macrophages diminish in numbers relative to other types of cells in the inflamed area.[13,201,202]

c. Fibroblasts in the interstices commence to grow rapidly, show experimental evidence of incorporation of DNA from lymphocytes, and [42,227,228] commence to deposit collagen in quantity.[13,201,202]

d. Lymphatics and blood vessels in the area commence to regenerate and link up with their counterparts in adjacent healthy tissue.[13,201,202]

e. Necrobiotic peripheral tissue cells and their residues vanish.[13,201,202]

f. Remaining healthy peripheral tissue cells, both in the damaged or grafted area and in adjacent healthy tissue, commence to grow rapidly and bridge the gap between healthy and damaged.[13,201,202]

g. Many of the peripheral tissue cells, whether they be within the adjacent healthy area or in a graft, will be found to contain disintegrating small lymphocytes and usually more than one normally expects to see in similar cells under normal conditions.[226]

h. The area commences to heal, gain tensile strength, and resume normal function at a rapid rate.[13,201,202]

The rate at which all the aforementioned events transpire is known to be slowed by lymphocytolytic agents, such as cortisol, and by drugs which interfere with nucleic acid synthesis, particularly in lymphocytes,[201,211] e.g. Purinethol,® Imuran® l-asparaginase, and methotrexate.

5. Recycling of Free Extracellular Proteins during Infection

Under conditions wherein pathogenic microorganisms are introduced, and depending somewhat on their pathogenicity (often dependent on the proteolitic effect of the free extracellular proteins produced), evidence for such cycling of proteins can be outlined as follows. First, in addition to peripheral (interstitial) microphagic and macrophagic phagocytosis of their free extracellular proteins or of the bacteria themselves—a process often destructive to the microphages or macrophages [13,201,202]—within a few hours the primary immunologic response commences in the regional nodes, as outlined in B, 1. Second, some six to ten days after their invasion (or injection), and if a successful immunologic response takes place, several events transpire almost simultaneously. Such events include all those described on pp. 233-246, with the variation that the bacteria, as well as the cells they have damaged, commence to vanish rapidly after the sixth to tenth day. While it remains to be demonstrated that the small lymphocytes returning from the lymphoid organs are directly responsible for bacterial lysis, the timing of bacterial disappearance in a successful primary immunologic response corresponds to this event, rather than to the humoral agglutinin response which usually occurs earlier, as emphasized by Lawrence.[187]

The lymphocytolytic drugs and all immunosuppressive measures to be described later delay a successful primary immunologic response. If the invading microorganism is a virus whose infectivity is primarily intracellular within peripheral tissue cells, the whole immune process may take longer, possibly owing to an initial delay in the production and excretion of abnormal proteins from peripheral tissue cells which they have invaded. Moreover, it is possible that in order to destroy the intracellular virus, the immune processes operative must also destroy some of the cells which the viruses have invaded, or repair their DNA.

6. Recycling of Free Extracellular Proteins during Allografting

Under conditions where genetically different (heterologous) grafts are applied, evidence for such recycling of proteins is quite clearly as follows. First, corresponding to the degree of histoincompatibility and to some extent to the intrinsic nature of lymphatic drainage in the area where the graft is applied, in addition to the microphagic (polymorphonuclear) and macrophagic disposition of debris from damaged cells grafted to the periphery, within a few hours the primary immunologic response takes place in the regional nodes.[202] The serial cellular responses are as listed pp. 233-240. Second, six to ten days after the grafting, and at the same time that newly informed (immunologically competent) small lymphocytes in the secondary follicles of lymphoid organs commence to migrate from their site of origin to the periphery, several events transpire almost simultaneously:

1. Small lymphocytes become the most numerous and prominent cells in the grafted area.[202]

2. Small lymphocytes directly induce lysis of the grafted cells.[96,202]

3. Macrophages and microphages again may become prominent cells surrounding the graft (presumably to reutilize the necrotic cellular debris).

4. Small lymphocytes continue to pour into the area, while fibroblasts and other regenerating tissue elements grow at an accelerated rate (to repair and heal the defect which will remain upon rejection of the graft).

Measures which delay rejection of the graft and subsequent healing of the isologous tissues include lymphocytolytic drugs such as cortisol, lymphocytolytic agents, and antilymphocyte serum; drugs which reduce DNA synthesis in lymphocytes, such as Purinethol, Imuran, etc.; neonatal thymectomy; diversion of thoracic duct lymph to the exterior (if the graft is below the diaphragm); local interruption of the afferent or efferent drainage of the regional nodes; and total-body or local radiation to destroy the lymphocytes. Such "immunosuppressive" measures are being explored singly or in combination currently to make the graft survive—*but possibly at the expense of the host* (see Chap. 19).

7. The Combined Trophic and Immunologic Significance of Recycling

Next, it is significant that in the framework of such sequential utilization and cycling of macromolecular substrate emanating from damaged cells, microorganisms, and grafted heterologous cells to the regional nodes, and from there via the circulation, there resides a mechanism not only for reutilizing the free extracellular proteins which they secrete but also for reutilizing them in a manner such that the plasma and small lymphocytes which return from the lymphoid organs will actually destroy the parasites from which the free extracellular proteins were secreted. The parasites, then, will be removed from a status where they are feeding on the cells and body fluids of the host and growing at his expense to a status where they are lysed and reutilized as substrate in a healthy host whose cells, particularly his lymphoid cells, grow at their expense. Moreover, via the information and substrate brought back to the peripheral tissues by increased quantities of circulating lymphocytes and plasma (owing to local hyperemia), healthy peripheral cells of the host can be stimulated to grow at an increased rate to repair the defect which remains following destruction of the parasites and the tissue cells which they have already destroyed. Thus one may look upon the immune reaction, the *host-parasite reaction* or the *host vs. graft reaction* as a sophisticated form of trophism in which lymphoid elements augment their feeding function of host cells by neutralizing (via antibodies) or lysing (via small lymphocytes) material which is genetically incompatible, foreign or spurious. As a result, this material is reduced to a form in which it can be reutilized conveniently and without toxicity for the nourishment of cells in the host.

Such considerations are entirely in accord with Lavoisier's principles of mass and energy conservation which state that matter cannot cease to exist but must be dissipated in one form or another into the medium wherein it is destroyed. Therefore, *immunity should be recognized not only as the power to destroy but also as the capacity to reutilize or excrete matter which is foreign.* Because the points of entry of foreign matter into multicellular organisms, such as humans, are usually at some distance from the usual points of excretion from the body, one must look toward reutilization, at least temporarily, as the primary method of dissipation or disposition. The regional nodes merely reside in a position admirably adapted to carry on a large share of the initial reutilization. But the kidneys ultimately must be expected to excrete the bulk of the residua, preferably in non-toxic forms.*

8. The Logistic and Genetic Significance of Reutilization and Recycling

It is significant in living individuals that in the sequential lymphoid cell reutilization, processing, and cycling of free extracellular proteins emanating *simultaneously* from healthy isologous cells, damaged isologous cells, microorganisms, and grafted foreign cells, there resides an effective mechanism whereby recognition codes in newly produced plasma proteins and circulating lymphocytes are adapted quite rapidly to recognize and react with foreign matter, while continuing to recognize and feed endogenous cells. Moreover, such reutilization, processing, and recycling will allow lymphoid elements to perform their useful functions without having to alter significantly the ambient rate of lymphopoiesis in organs other than the regional nodes. Such considerations are cogent from a purely logistic point of view, for if the migration of newly formed plasma and circulating lymphocytes is random through the vascular system and intravascular mixing is efficient, relatively large quantities of both must be maintained to mount an effective immunologic response in any given tissue supplied by a segment of the vascular system, while relatively large quantities must remain to continue their feeding function throughout remaining body tissues supplied by the vascular system as a whole.

With respect to quantitatively significant adaptation of recognition codes in the plasma proteins and in the DNA of circulating lymphocytes, the relatively small quantity of free extracellular proteins emanating from damaged isologous cells, microorganisms, and grafted cells, initially processed in given regional nodes, then recycled to remaining lymphoid organs, would seem very important. With respect to maintenance of the capacity to recognize and nourish self, the relatively large quan-

---

*If reutilization is incomplete, one may find deposition of antigen-antibody compexes or amyloid in the germinal centers, spleen, liver, or kidneys (see pp. 239 and 240).

tities of free extracellular proteins emanating from healthy cells throughout the body, initially processed in many regional nodes, and recycled to be reutilized in all lymphoid organs, including those regional to sites of tissue damage or infection, would seem very important. With respect to maintenance of stability in ambient rates of lymphopoiesis throughout the lymphoid organs, the relatively large mass of healthy isologous cells giving rise to free extracellular proteins, as compared with the mass of physiologically altered or damaged cells, microorganisms, or grafted cells doing so under relatively normal conditions, would seem important.

It may follow then that the free extracellular proteins emanating from healthy isologous cells all over the body help to stabilize the DNA in developing small lymphocytes so that they maintain the capacity for self-recognition and self-nourishment. On the other hand, the DNA donated to peripheral tissue cells via small lymphocytes stabilizes or supplements peripheral cell DNA in directing local growth and differention. Through stabilization of lymphocytic DNA by appropriate donations from many peripheral cells to the nodes, circulation of nodal proteins and lymphocytes to all lymphoid organs, and appropriate donations of DNA from many lymphoid organs via lymphoctyes to the periphery, the heritable, inherent, genetic characteristics of the species, the individual within the species, and the cells of the individual may remain relatively stable under a wide variety of conditions, including physical damage, infection, and allografting (provided doses of the latter are not overwhelming [229]) .

Such considerations are cogent because they may help explain:

1. Why in tissue culture systems, lacking the cycling of free extracellular proteins from healthy isologous peripheral cells to lymphoid organs and lacking the recycling of small lymphocytes and plasma from multiple lymphoid organs to the cells growing in the artificial medium, the small lymphocytes appear to lose their characteristic differentiated appearance to resemble blast cells; take on features characteristic of embryonal or malignant cells, including active (uncontrolled?) RNA synthesis, protein production, anaerobic glycolysis; and thus grow to lack several

of the features characteristic of small lymphocytes in the body.

2. Why therapeutic measures killing relatively large numbers of small lymphocytes are prone to be associated with undesirable side effects such as wasting or a greatly increased incidence of malignancy (see Chap. 19 and Reference 230).

3. Why in chronic lymphocytic leukemia, a disease in which many, if not most, of the circulating lymphocytes appear abnormal, there appears to be an unusually high incidence of wasting, abnormal immunologic reactions, or malignancy in other tissues, either singly or in combination.[231]

4. Why genetic engineering through injections of foreign proteins, RNA, or DNA may prove relatively ineffective and not without unexpected side effects in living individuals owing to the relatively great individuality and mass and to the relatively rapid processing and recycling in the individual's pool of corresponding compounds.

Such considerations on the simultaneous recognition of living matter which is foreign or diseased and that which is endogenous and healthy are in accordance with the *"immunologic surveillance"* concept of Burnet.[198] However, my concept differs in that it places the emphasis on how recognition takes place through serial processing in heterogeneous mononuclear cells, rather than by clonal selection in mutant lymphocytes whose random genetic mutations not only remain to be observed in healthy individuals but also are just as likely to be unselective, aberrant, or disadvantageous. Moreover, it takes into account how the mononuclear cells and the free extracellular proteins to which they give rise are dissipated during health (whether or not a definitive immunologic challenge is present) instead of hiding in clones waiting for an appropriate antigen or another exposure to a similar antigen, and in clones which must be calculated to almost infinite in number if all potential antigens encountered during a lifetime are to be covered.

9. Morphostasis

Thus far we have considered only the consequences of sequential lymphoid cellular utilization and cycling of proteins which emanate from "healthy isologous cells," as well as from physically damaged isologous cells, microorganisms, and grafted heterologous cells. Even more subtle may be the consequences of physiologic changes which undoubtedly take place in "healthy isologous cells" as the result of changing but tolerable environmental influences such as temperature, diet, and atmospheric conditions, which necessitate the performance of genetically inherited functions at accelerated or decelerated rates. Burwell [232] has proposed that small lymphocytes can modulate the functions performed by other kinds of cells in the body via immunologic mechanisms involving surface antigen-antibody reactions. He has suggested that such a modulatory role of the lymphocytes is normally in the direction of maintaining homeostasis and has therefore defined the role of the lymphocytes as being *morphostatic*.

Such a concept has great theoretical importance, but if the foregoing interpretations of observations are correct, the morphostatic role of the small lymphocytes must be expected to penetrate well beyond the cell surface to the very heart or nucleus of the cell which the small lymphocyte is capable of invading and to which it may donate its DNA. Similarly, the complicated sequential cellular route by which proteins secreted from peripheral tissue cells are transferred and subsequently reutilized to pass information on to the nucleus of the small lymphocyte must be expected to go deeper than the surface of intermediary cells.

Focussing on the regional nodes, then, one may envision morphostatic organs specialized to utilize substrate, information, and energy from two sources (a) arterial blood which carries in quantities of oxygen, water, salts, glucose, amino acids, fats, plasma proteins, and formed elements, including lymphocytes circulated from other hemopoietic organs and (b) peripheral lymph which carries in proteins and other molecules excreted from peripheral tissue cells (and often from microbes) and which also carries in relatively small quantities of plasma and formed elements exuded from the peripheral arteriovenous capillaries. Aliquots from (a) are utilized for growth and differentiation in relatively homogeneous populations of mononuclear cells, such as large, medium-sized, and small lymphocytes, surrounding the arterioles in the cortical portions of the nodes. Residual aliquots from (a) and aliquots from (b) are utilized for growth and differentiation in heterogeneous populations of mononuclear cells, such as histiocytes, macrophages, monocytes, plasmacytes, and medium-sized lymphocytes surrounding the sinusoids in the medullary portions. The latter cell populations are especially oriented to reutilize free extracellular proteins, especially antigenic ones, emanating from the periphery to produce modified free extracellular proteins which, upon circulation from the medullary areas into the systemic circulation and on to diverse lymphoid organs, may modify informational codes in the DNA of small lymphocytes produced in the cortical areas of many. The last, upon migrating via the circulation from the cortical areas of each to medullary areas and from there onward via the systemic circulation to other lymphoid and nonlymphoid organs, may donate their DNA genetically intact to recipient cells. Reutilizing this DNA, the recipient cells in all areas may be kept informed in a manner appropriate to the benefit of all, regardless of their exact location.

10. Summary in Perspective

Correlating the foregoing, one may conceive of the lymphoid tissue mass as an integrated system of cells whose purpose is to feed and be fed by diverse peripheral tissue cells. The lymphoid tissue mass grows and must learn to do so with increasing efficiency, the larger and more complicated the body becomes. Since information is a prerequisite to learning, the concerted activity of lymphoid tissue cells is to reutilize and integrate information, along with substrate emanating from diverse peripheral cells so that appropriate forms of substrate will be fed back to peripheral cells via the circulating plasma and circulating mononuclear cells to which the many lymphoid organs give rise. Relatively large quantities of genetic material in the form of DNA, are indigenous to the system and serve as the template upon which incoming information is transcribed through the serial action of multiple definitive types of mononuclear lymphoid cells. Upon imprintation, this DNA serves as the mold from which large quantities of outgoing information are patterned to seek out appropriate binding sites in the peripheral cells. Through feedback of such coded information, along with various forms of substrate, the growth and function of peripheral tissue cells may be governed as well as nurtured under normal and abnormal conditions.

Under obviously abnormal conditions when damaged cells, microorganisms, or foreign cells are growing in the body and therefore presenting information and substrate foreign to the system, the lymphoid tissue mass, upon recycling free extracellular proteins from the latter, may feed back modified free extracellular proteins and DNA within small migratory lymphocytes repectively coded to agglutinate or destroy the spurious or obnoxious sources of this information and substrate. As a result, such foreign sources and their free extracellular proteins may be reduced into nontoxic forms which can be reutilized conveniently for growth and continuing function in healthy cells of the host.

Although the lymphoid tissue mass in all multicellular organisms appears oriented toward performing similar functions, in very complicated organisms, such as air-breathing vertebrates, the thymus and small cytoplasm-poor lymphocytes grow and specialize out of the mass to accelerate and implement the efficiency with which essential trophic and immunologic functions are performed by the mass as a whole.

C. THE ACQUISITION AND DONATION OF ENERGY ALONG WITH SUBSTRATE AND INFORMATION

To synthesize complicated proteins, to grow, to differentiate, to move, to feed, to destroy, and to do all in superlative fashion, requires superlative energy. Although in mammalian cells, energy is ultimately derived primarily from the aerobic oxidation of glucose, it is normally transferred and stored in the form of phosphate reversibly linked to nucleosides, such as purine (e.g. adenosine) or pyrimidines (e.g. thymidine), whose linked forms or nucleotides (ATP, ADP, AMP, and TPN-DPN-MPN) contain phosphate bonds capable of high-energy yield upon hydrolysis in the aqueous internal environment.[233,234] Therefore, the following facts are significant. First, the lymphoid organs, particularly the thymus, contain the highest concentrations of nucleoside-bound phosphate in the body, as is evidenced by analysis for DNA bound phosphorous (see Introduction and Tables VI–VIII). Second, the lymphoid organs also contain relatively high concentrations of phosphate bound to the nucleosides of RNA, as is estimated by direct measurement of RNA-bound phosphorous (RNA-P). Moreover, they differ from remaining organs containing relatively high RNA-P concentrations, such as the pancreas, salivary glands, and liver, in that they secrete their cytoplasmic products into the vascular system instead of into the gastrointestinal tract. Third, they turn over their nucleosides and their phosphorous relatively rapidly in comparison with remaining body tissues, as is estimated by their rate of incorporation of $^{32}PO_4$, ^3HT, tritiated adenosine, tritiated uridine, or tritiated cytidine (the latter indicating rapid RNA synthesis).[235] Finally, they appear well supplied with oxygen and glucose, as evidenced by their superlative arterial circulation as described in Section one and p. 171-178).

It is therefore necessary to consider briefly how this energy may be dissipated from the lymphoid organs and reutilized elsewhere. Under relatively normal conditions and in decremental order as a function of time, dissipation may proceed as follows.

In the plasma. Having utilized energy to synthesize cytoplasm, several types of lymphoid cells may dissipate it by shedding cytoplasm to produce plasma (see Chap. 9). This plasma, upon leaving the lymphoid organs to enter the circulation, contains free extracellular proteins whose colloid osmotic energy[225,236] balances the force of hydrostatic pressure within the vascular system and thus enables the circulating blood to retain water on the intravascular side of semipermeable (capillary) membranes. Until such time as these free extracellular proteins break down or leave the vascular system to give up their substance (and their energy) to other cells, their colloid osmotic energy continues as an important force within the intravascular compartment.

As the plasma proteins break down (as we know they must by their relatively short biologic lives),[166] one may expect that the energy of peptide bonds [233] will be released along with the amino acids which result from the breakdown of proteins. One can only presume that these breakdown products will become available to tissues in general. With respect to the differential utilization of "normal plasma proteins" versus antibody proteins, it may be suspected but not proven that both can be utilized in other tissues via the same pathways. This is true particularly if we consider that antibodies merely represent terminal molecular modifications on normal plasma proteins.[196a,b,197]

For lack of knowledge, the energy potentially expended by antibodies and by complement in binding antigens will not be discussed, although it would seem likely that exergonic reactions are involved.

In small cytoplasm-poor lymphocytes. Having utilized energy to synthesize nucleoplasm and cytoplasm, and having shed most of their cytoplasm during the course of differentiation (see Chap. 9), small cytoplasm-poor lymphocytes are shed from the lymphoid organs into the circulation. Energy contained in their nucleoplasm and relatively scant cytoplasm will be shed with them. The small lymphocytes, then, may continue to expend energy as follows:

1. By moving actively and at an exceedingly rapid rate against the resistance imposed by solid tissues which they invade upon leaving the vascular system. It is of significance here that the small cytoplasm-poor lymphocytes are relatively lacking in mitochondria [127,237] and therefore presumably obtain energy for movement from other internal sources rather than from the aerobic oxidation of glucose and oxidative phosphorylations within a relatively tiny mitochondrial mass.[127]

2. By entering other tissue cells, disintegrating, and giving up their energy as well as other components to the tissue cells which they have invaded. As pointed out by Kelsall,[10] this energy may enhance the reutilization of substrate for protein synthesis in the invaded cells.

3. By disintegrating in the plasma or in the interstices to give

up their energy and their substance for purposes which remain to be determined.[9]

4. By undergoing explosive lysis upon contacting or entering an isologous cell recognized as being incompatible, or upon contacting (or entering) a foreign cell recognized as being genetically incompatible. The latter type of lymphocyte disintegration, as observed in tissue cultures by Sherwin,[144] results not only in lysis of the lymphocytes but also in the explosive lysis of the cell contacted or entered. This explosive form of lysis, somewhat reminiscent of an atomic chain reaction, seems particularly important in that it indicates from where the energy is derived, upon recognition, to lyse effete isologous cells or genetically incompatible foreign cells and thus reduce the latter into forms of substrate which can be reutilized conveniently.

Under abnormal conditions, particularly during stress, it is characteristic of the lymphocytes, particularly the small lymphocytes, in the thymus and remaining lymphoid organs to undergo lysis *in situ*, i.e. before they have migrated from the lymphoid organs as intact cells.[2-5,9,10,12,13,56] The small lymphocytes throughout the thymic cortex and those surrounding the germinal centers of the secondary lymph follicles in remaining lymphoid organs undergo lysis earlier and more extensively than those in the medullary areas.[2,9,10,12,15,56] As a result of this lymphocytolysis, mediated by adrenal glucose-active steroids,[12,56,132,133] the lymphoid tissue mass throughout the body is dissipated and shrinks suddenly. The thymus shrinks most rapidly, probably owing to its relatively great concentration of small cytoplasm-poor lymphocytes. As the small lymphocytes disintegrate and the lymphoid tissues shrink correspondingly, it follows that the circulating body fluids and secondarily the tissues become the potential recipients of increased quantities of small lymphocyte substance, an important constituent of which is nucleoplasm, hence DNA. As a relatively high concentration of nucleoside-bound phosphate is present in DNA, it follows, then, that increased amounts of nucleoside-bound phosphorous are being made available for some purpose. Noting, finally, that tissue anoxia is a common denominator of stress [12] and that an adequate physiologic response to stress connotes

in severa
suddenly
phate b(
energy.
aerobic
pensated
action,
charge o
Such
teries ir
but also
nucleosi
they ma
informa
strate w
may be
batterie
vasculai
must b
systems

D. '
A

The
only a
well as
atively
animal
relativ(
degree
in tim(
and p1
rioven
fore th
per u1
immec
comes
poor l

a capacity to expend extraordinary energy (effort), it follows that one of the physiologic purposes of stress lymphocytolysis is to increase the quantity of nucleoside-bound (high-energy) phosphate available for reutilization in the tissues under conditions when energy available from aerobic oxidation of glucose is in relatively short supply.

Theoretically, this form of energy, particularly that which may result from lymphocytolysis in the thymus, would seem most relevant at the time of birth when the thymus is largest relative to body size and then commences its involution at the same time that the newborn must start to search on his own for food in a relatively hostile extra uterine environment with weak muscles, partially expanded lungs, and anoxic tissues. It is important then that the energy necessary for muscle contraction is obtained by transfer of phosphate from adenosine (ATP) to creatine, thus creating phosphocreatine from which the energy for contraction is derived directly.[225,233]

It may follow that the failure of the thymus to undergo involution and release such nucleoside-bound phosphate energy is an important pathogenic factor in sudden unexplained death and in crib death. These catastrophic diseases are characterized by little evidence of agonal struggle (muscle contraction), relatively minimal cause for anoxia, and a thymus which has failed to undergo expected age involution or a thymus which has not undergone involution and remains fused to the parathyroid glands (which are also critically involved in the metabolism of phosphate).[238,239]

In myasthenia gravis, one sees a somewhat similar disease, wherein the thymus often remains relatively or grossly enlarged, the muscles unexplainably become weak, and the individual dies, usually of anoxia owing to paralysis of the respiratory muscles or paralysis of the pharyngeal muscles (which results in aspiration pnuemonitis). One may speculate, therefore, that myasthenia gravis represents chronic failure to release or transfer nucleotide, nucleic acid, or nuclear power during stress from the thymus to muscles, particularly the muscles concerned with respiration and swallowing. Unexplained sudden and crib death represent

to naturally occurring diseases has filled many texts and will continue to do so because the precise etiologic agents and their way of operating remain elusive. In other words, we often cannot explain what is happening in the individual's unsuccessful fight to devour an agent which is attempting to devour him.

In order to gain additional clinical insight into the normal and abnormal responses of the lymphatic apparatus, it is necessary, therefore, to turn to iatrogenic (physician-produced) diseases wherein the pathogens are known, carefully selected, administered in known quantity to specific body sites, and observed under variable but carefully controlled conditions. Most of the latter criteria are met in the clinical and experimental study of the graft rejection phenomenon. Some of the pertinent findings from these forms of study may be summarized as follows.

In healthy animals and humans wherein a state of homeostasis is presumed to exist, rejection of heterologous skin grafts commences at 7 to 10 days and is usually complete at 14 days. The usual reactions in the regional nodes and some of the small lymphocyte reactions toward the graft are outlined in Chapter 18, B.

In all species, grafts from closely related syngeneic donors survive somewhat longer and appear to function better than grafts from unrelated donors of the same species. Grafts from other species thus far have survived and functioned relatively poorly.[244] Such observations indicate that genetic similarity is important to prolonged graft survival (and may well be important to the prolonged survival of certain pathogenic and nonpathogenic microorganisms in the body).

In general, allografts from areas where lymphathic drainage is poor normally, usually survive somewhat longer than skin allografts. Moreover, skin allografts to skin pedicles suspended from the host solely by afferent arteries and veins, i.e. with peripheral lymphatics divided, usually survive for prolonged periods of time [245] (usually until the peripheral lymphatics regenerate). Such findings emphasize the importance of the peripheral or "afferent limb" of the lymphatic apparatus in the rejection phenomenon. These findings also give some indication as to why renal allografts often survive longer than conventional allografts (perhaps owing to the fact that the bulk of the graft is suspended from the host on a similar pedicle).

The survival of allografts, irrespective of kind and species, is greatly enhanced by "immunosuppressive measures" directed toward reducing the number of small lymphocytes in the circulating blood which may ultimately return (at random) to the graft site.[244]

A. IMMUNOSUPPRESSIVE MEASURES
a. Neonatal Thymectomy in Experimental Animals and Thymectomy Prior to Grafting in Adult Animals

Neonatal thymectomy has proven effective in experimental animals, but if the young animal is tolerant to an allograft, he usually succumbs from "runt disease," a disease characterized by failure to grow at a normal rate, generalized atrophy of the lymphoid tissues (including intestinal lymphoid tissue), and increased susceptibility to infection, diarrhea, and death, praticularly if he continues to live in the ambient environment.[19-21,23-26,63] In neonatally thymectomized animals without allografts, the same disease usually supervenes in free living animals, indicating that the disease is owing to neonatal thymectomy, and not to the allograft, by itself.[19] A germ-free environment prevents this disease, but the growth rate remains retarded and the lymphoid tissues usually appear relatively atrophic,[64-68] indicating that the thymus and the lymphoid tissues normally supply something besides immunologic protection to remaining body tissues. Thymectomy during adult life, on the other hand, is not associated with such complications but does not significantly prolong allograft survival. (The theoretical reasons for all these findings are discussed in terms of mass action in Chap 15.)

b. Total Body Irradiation

This method of immunosuppression is based on the observation that lymphocytes, particularly small lymphocytes, are approximately ten times as radiosensitive as most remaining body cells [127] and predicated on the assumption that radiation doses

can be achieved which will destroy all or most of the lymphocytes but be relatively harmless to remaining cells in the body.
Under ambient atmospheric conditions (20% oxygen, 760 mm
Hg barometric pressure) 500 rads total body radiation is a median
lethal dose which will destroy all of the small lymphocytes and
most of the medium-sized lymphocytes in the body and which will
produce acute radiation sickness, a disease characterized by profound lymphoid tissue atrophy throughout all lymphoid tissues
(including the intestine), anorexia, nausea, vomiting, diarrhea,
lack of resistance to infection, and death (more or less in this
order).[246] Approximately one half the animals or humans thus
irradiated will die within 10 to 14 days [246] unless some of the
hematopoietic organs (e.g. spleen or bone marrow) are shielded
at the time of irradiation or unless they are given transfusions of
bone marrow [23] (containing stromal, as well as cellular elements;
see Chap. 16, B). Depending on the dosage chosen (e.g. 500–5000
rads but usually 1000–2000 rads; see Chap.4), the shielded area
may prove effective in repopulating both the unshielded lymphoid and myeloid organs of the individuals.[23,246,247] If splenic
or marrow transfusions are given instead of shielding, depending on the volume of tissue given and the radiation dosage, the
cells from an unrelated donor may effectively repopulate the
bone marrow of the host, grow there, and produce erythrocytes,
granulocytes, and platelets resembling those of the donor, which
will circulate in the host, allowing him to survive much longer
than 10 to 14 days.[23] Under the latter circumstances, the bone
marrow graft will continue to produce donor-type cells, but the
lymphoid organs remain atrophic and the host usually succumbs
from a "graft vs. host reaction." This is a disease characterized
by generalized lymphoid tissue atrophy (including the lymphoid
tissue of the small intestine), failure to grow at a normal rate,
anorexia, increased susceptibility to infection, and death.[23] On
the other hand, if the lymphoid organs become repopulated with
lymphoid cells, particularly medium- and small-sized lymphocytes,
the bone marrow graft is rejected and the body becomes repopulated with blood cells of the host type [23] (provided he has survived
both irradiation and this form of allografting). The hazards

involved in this form of immunosuppression have generally precluded its clinical use, except in inadvertent radiation exposure in radiation laboratories, even though the host may be tolerant to another tissue of the same donor or another donor during the period the marrow allograft is thriving.[23]

c. Local Body Irradiation

This form of immunosuppression is based on the premise that if the small lymphocytes formed in nodes regional to the graft can be effectively destroyed by proper administration and timing of irradiation, the graft-rejection phenomenon can be prevented. Also, if the graft site is included in the radiation field, the premise continues that the small lymphocytes returning to the graft may be destroyed. Local irradiation thus far has proved relatively ineffective for the following theoretical reasons. First, the doses between 500 and 2000 rads used to destroy the lymphocytes do not effectively destroy the relatively radioinsensitive histiocytes, macrophages, plasmacytes, and reticular cells in the regional nodes [96,246] and (over the period of study) do not greatly affect the small lymphocytes growing in more distant lymphoid organs which may receive combinations of substrate and information (antigen-antibody complexes or altered proteins?) disseminated from the histiocytes, macrophages, and plasmacytes into the circulation via efferent regional nodal lymph (see Chap. 18, B). Second, sufficient radiation to continually kill the small lymphocytes returning to the graft site from many different distant lymphoid organs will ultimately be damaging to the graft.

d. Extracorporeal Radiation of Blood (or Lymph)

This method immunosuppression is based on the observation that small lymphocytes are exceedingly radiosensitive in comparison with remaining blood elements [127,246,248-250] and the assumption (possibly) that a large proportion of the small lymphocytes have a prolonged total lifespan (e.g. 100 days), a prolonged recirculation in the vascular system from lymph to blood and back to lymph (e.g. 100 days; see Chap. 16, E). Therefore there is an opportunity for most to pass through the extracorporeal circuit where the radiation is delivered. However, if the lifespan of the majority of small lymphocytes is relatively short (e.g. 2 days) and their intravascular lifespan very short (e.g. 2 hours) as they pass from lymph to blood on their way to other tissues (see Chap. 16, E, 3), and as their high order of radiation sensitivity would suggest*, many can be expected to bypass the extracorporeal circuit on their way from the lymphoid organs to the tissues. In calves, extracorporeal radiation of blood (or lymph) has proven to be an effective means of immunosuppression, as evidenced by prolongation of graft tolerance. However, as with total-body irradiation, the lymphoid organs become atrophic, some of the animals fail to grow at a normal rate, and they demonstrate increased susceptibility to infection.[248] In humans, the technology involved and the time spent tied up to the machine have precluded widespread application and evaluation of the method as a single form of immunosuppression,[249] but development of smaller portable beta-emitting devices appears imminent.[250] At tolerable dosage levels, extracorporeal irradiation of blood has been found to be very effective in producing profound lymphocytopenia [248] and has been found to be a useful means of producing hematologic remission in certain forms of leukemia.[249,250] While the method has shown considerable promise as a temporary adjunct to other immunosuppressive regimens, it appears to carry with it the same inherent complications as total-body irradiation when used alone in doses sufficient to produce prolonged graft tolerance, at least in calves.[248]

It is significant to reiterate here that small cytoplasm-poor lymphocytes, such as those found in the peripheral blood and in the mantle zones of secondary lymph follicles, not only contain a relatively high cellular concentration of DNA and a relatively high concentration of phosphate bound to the nucleosides of their DNA, and turn over the phosphate in their DNA relatively rapidly (as measured by rates of $^{32}PO_4$ incorporation as compared with nonlymphoid cells) but also that they are the most radiosensitive cells in the body.[127,246] It appears that the nucleoside-

---

*The radiation sensitivity of body cells in general is inversely proportional to their lifespan and directly proportional to their rate of growth.[127]

phosphate bonds in their DNA are highly radiosensitive targets, being partially split by as little as 50 rads of radiation in an animal respiring under atmospheric conditions (see Chap. 2). Moreover, their rate of complete lysis, both within the lymphoid organs and in the blood, is so rapid after doses of 500 rads [12,127,246] that it must be assumed their nucleoside-phosphate bond energy resides in relatively unstable form. Such instability may be an important factor not only in the radiation sensitivity of lymphocytes, but also in the capacity of the small lymphocytes (upon recognition) * to lyse other cells to which they have become sensitized (see Chap. 18, C).

e. Radioactive Isotopes Bound to Compounds

While $^{32}PO_4$ or ^{3}HT, owing to their high initial rate of incorporation into lymphoid organs and lymphocytes, at first glance might appear to be ideal agents to carry ionizing radiation preferentially to lymphocytes, the subsequent uptake of $^{32}PO_4$ in areas where phosphate concentration is higher but turnover slower (as in bones) precludes the immunosuppressive use of this compound of radioactive phosphorous whose biologic half-life is 14 days.[251] The prolonged half-life of tritium (12.1 years), the ultimate distribution of tritiated thymidine to nonlymphoid as well as lymphoid tissues whose growth rate is relatively rapid, and the ultimate dilution of breakdown products into body water still containing tritium [252] would seem to preclude the prolonged immunosuppressive use of ^{3}HT (whose usage in trace amounts has yielded so much valuable information concerning the growth rate of body cells in general). On the positive side, the ultimate concentration of $^{32}PO_4$ within bone and the fact that it is a good beta emitter while it is decaying have made this radioactive

---

* The process of recognition very recently has been shown by Andersson *et al.*[273] to involve a decrease in stability of phosphate bonds in DNA or desoxyribonucleoproteins, as is reflected by increased affinity toward basic dyes such as acridine orange, and during lymphocyte transformation induced by HL-A antigens (and by phytohemagglutinin). Noting that lysis in some lymphocytes and assumption of anaerobic respiration in others occur simultaneously with transformation, one wonders if the mutagen (or mitogen) may not be killing some lymphocytes, while rendering others malignant by paralyzing respiration (cf. Warburg [274]).

compound an ideal agent for treating myeloproliferative disorders such as chronic granulocytic leukemia and polycythemia
vera.[253,254] The clinical usage of $^{32}PO_4$ in lymphoproliferative disorders such as chronic lymphocytic leukemia [255] apparently has
not been in dosages sufficient to result in immunosuppression to
the degree that the patient under treatment will accept allografts without excessive radiation to the bone marrow concomi-
tantly.

Radioactive isotopes of iodine bound to colloids or oils such
as lipiodal, may have theoretical usage in immunosuppression, particularly when injected into regional lymphatics to be
carried to regional nodes. The clinical usage of such radioactive
compounds in the treatment of metastatic disease in the regional
lymph nodes is under active study. Insufficient data has accumulated to warrant its discussion as an immunosuppressive measure.

f. Radiomimetic Drugs

An outgrowth of the development of mustard gases for chemical
warfare during World War I was the clinical application of alkylating agents such as nitrogen mustard, TEM, chlorambucil,
busulfan, and thio-tepa.[251] Such chemical compounds, especially
nitrogen mustard and chlorambucil, proved to be radiomi-
metic in many of their cytotoxic actions, particularly with respect
to producing appreciable sudden lymphocytolysis throughout the
lymphoid organs and in suppressing immunologic reactions.[251]
It is significant in view of earlier considerations that the cytotoxic
action of these drugs appears to be primarily on nucleoproteins
through clumping or crosslinking the macromolecules in DNA,
probably as the result of esterification of phosphate groupings.[251]
The relatively great cytotoxic action on lymphocytes may well be
due to the relatively high concentration of DNA and DNA-bound
phosphate in lymphocytes (as compared with other body cells).
Such drugs have proven to be particularly useful in the treatment
of malignant lymphomas and are also good but relatively unselective immunosuppressants. Their clinical usage as immunosuppressants has been hampered by the fact that a relatively narrow
margin exists between immunosuppresive and toxic doses.[225] The

signs and symptoms of toxicity again include nausea, vomiting, diarrhea, rapid wasting, profound lymphocytopenia in the lymphoid organs and blood, desquamation of the small intestinal mucosa, pancytopenia, increased susceptibility to infection, and death [251] (more or less in this order as a function of time after a lethal dose). It is of possible significance, finally, that although chlorambucil is absorbed by the small intestinal mucosa and therefore can be expected to attain a relatively high concentration during absorption in this radiosensitive tissue, massive desquamation of the mucosa seems to await generalized lymphocytolysis and lymphocytopenia.[251]

g. *Drugs Interfering with DNA Synthesis in Lymphocytes*

Since the rate of DNA synthesis is relatively great in lymphocytes as compared with that in remaining cells of the body, it should be possible theoretically to find analogues of DNA precursors which will compete with, or drugs which will retard, DNA production in lymphocytes without significantly retarding DNA synthesis in remaining body cells; or to find certain drugs which will specifically interfere with information codes in lymphocyte DNA such that lymphocytes cannot recognize and destroy other cells. An active search by researchers throughout the world continues for such ideal immunosuppressives. Drugs which have been synthesized (or recovered from bacteria) in this category include Purinethol, Imuran, methotrexate, L-asparaginase, and many others.[251]

Imuran (azothioprine), a conjugated derivative of purinethol (6-mercaptopurine) has been found to be relatively efficacious[251] and at present constitutes one of the mainstays of prolonged immunosuppressive regimens to prevent the rejection of human allografts.[244] This drug and its analogue, purinethol, appear to interfere specifically with interconversion of nucleotides (nucleosides bound to phosphorous) in DNA, thus retarding DNA synthesis [251]—a finding which again points toward the importance of the high-energy phosphate bond in DNA (see Chap. 18, C). At dosage levels which are both tolerable and clinically immunosuppressive, Imuran and the remaining drugs in this category produce variable but relatively uniform lymphocytopenia throughout the lymphoid organs and in the blood.[251] In toxic or lethal doses, they produce profound lymphocytopenia in the lymphoid organs and in the blood, together with nausea, vomiting, diarrhea, sloughing of the intestinal mucosa, increased susceptibility to infection, and death (more or less in the same order as a function of time).[251] In therapeutic, but nonlethal doses, the prolonged use of these drugs along with other measures (e.g. cortisol) have been found to be associated with an increased susceptibility to infection,[244] a 200-fold increase in the expected rate of malignancy [244] (lymphoid, as well as nonlymphoid), and an accelerated incidence of inflammatory or degenerative vascular lesions, particularly in vessels feeding the graft.[256,257] By themselves and at tolerable dosage levels, none of these drugs used alone has been found to be satisfactorily immunosuppressive without some of the aforementioned complications, singly or in combination.[244]

Of theoretical and practical interest, of course, are the accelerated rates of development of malignancies and of arterial lesions which occur with the use of these immunosuppressive agents. In terms of preceding considerations (Chap. 16, C and 18, B), the increased incidence of malignant cellular proliferation perhaps can be explained by the lack of DNA returned to peripheral cells by decreased numbers of circulating lymphocytes, such that peripheral cell DNA is not stabilized in the face of chromosomal damage produced by the immunosuppressive agent (to which growing peripheral cells are only somewhat less sensitive than growing lymphocytes, e.g. by a factor of $1/10-1/100$). An additional factor may be that insufficient small lymphocytes return to given areas to lyse enough damaged or mutant cells.

The arterial lesions can perhaps be explained by the fact that there is a more rapid rate of sensitization of lymphocytes toward cells making up the vessels of an allograft than toward the parenchymal cells which it contains. As a result, the graft is rejected by having its blood supply cut off, instead of by having the bulk of its cells killed directly. This type of hypersensitivity reaction may be particularly important in the rejection of bulky grafts wherein the rate of growth (or turnover) of parenchymal cells is relatively slow, as in heart or liver allografts. An additional factor with respect to arterial lesions in bulky allografts may be that such grafts are attached and suspended in the recipient through their arteries and veins. Therefore, one may expect lymphatic regeneration (hence, establishment of continuity in the afferent limb of the rejection phenomenon) to occur first in relation to the vessels.

h. Cortisol and Adrenal Glucocorticoids

In the mid-1940's, when it was found that alkylating agents such as nitrogen mustard could be turned toward clinical rather than bellicose usage and before drugs interfering with DNA synthesis were actively being sought and tested, White and Dougherty [56,132,133] found, and Selye [12] emphasized, that a very potent lymphocytolytic agent is to be found in cortisol. This is a compound which occurs naturally in the body and one which is released in increased amounts during stress. While it remains to be determined how cortisol (first isolated in crystalline form by Kendall in 1933 and tested on patients by Hench in 1948 [258]) actually induces lysis in lymphoid cells, particularly in small lymphocytes and what ultimately happens to the products of their lysis under various conditions, including stress, exogenously administered cortisol and its purified or synthetic derivatives have proven to be foremost among the "wonder drugs"* of the 1950's and 1960's. Aside from their "antiinflammatory effects," these steroids have proven to be the second mainstay or backstay without which the remaining immunosuppressive measures usually falter [244] like a mast before the wind. The staying effect of cortisol perhaps is owing to the consideration that the products of lymphocytolysis are not irreparably damaged and therefore may be reutilized to advantage. Alone, as an immunosuppressive agent, cortisol has proven a clinical failure insofar as the prolonged acceptance of allografts is concerned.[244] Moreover, perhaps as a result of the lysis of small lymphocytes before they can migrate from the lymphoid organs, the clinical usage of cortisol

---

* "They are wonder drugs" in that they produce wonderful remissions in many diseases of obscure etiology and in that many are still wondering how and why they actually do so (see p. 413) .

phocyte sera as an ideal immunosuppressive therapy remains to be proven, their experimental use has proven to be an extremely valuable tool for investigation.[263]

k. Desensitization

As all of the aforementioned immunosuppressive measures, singly and in combination, have not proven fully effective in surmounting the "transplantation barrier," immunologists are turning at present toward intensive exploration of the possibility that ideal graft tolerance can be achieved if the precise antigens emanating from tissues to be grafted can be isolated and used to desensitize the individuals intended to receive grafts.[244] Such exploration, along with continued exploration of the measures already mentioned, undoubtedly will lead to a better understanding of how antigens, antibodies, and cells interact. Whether or not such exploration results in achievement of the "ideal" in graft tolerance, better understanding of the individual's reactions to naturally occurring diseases will follow.

As already suggested by Loutit,[266] items such as (a) through (k) support the thesis that the function of small lymphocytes is trophic as well as immunologic. In other words, these cells normally feed other cells in the body, as well as affording them immunologic protection by various mechanisms. Evidence has been presented that via their relatively generous supply of nuclear DNA, the small cytoplasm-poor lymphocytes feed relatively small quantities of valuable molecular substrate, relatively important forms of information, and unknown quantities of highly concentrated energy to healthy, rapidly growing cells. Moreover, evidence has been presented to indicate that via their DNA, they supply not only the information to recognize but also the bioenergetic power to destroy or lyse cells and other living organisms which are foreign, genetically incompatible, or spurious. If enough small lymphocytes or enough of their desoxyribonucleic acids are destroyed by radiologic or other chemotherapeutic measures, both the feeding and the immunologic function are destroyed more or less simultaneously, as is reflected in growth failure, wasting, lack of thrift, runting, secondary disease, or whatever one chooses to call the syndrome which usually accompanies immunosuppression in young, rapidly growing animals.* With prolonged immunosuppression in adults, a related phenomenon may be manifest in the accelerated development of malignancies which compete very successfully with healthy cells for substrate and thus engender wasting in the healthy ones. From a clinical point of view, it follows, therefore, that in selecting patients for grafting or for immunosuppressive treatment of naturally occurring diseases, the predicted outcome of the natural disease necessitating such vigorous forms of treatment must be weighed carefully against the complications which will arise as a result of such treatment.

---

* It should be noted that the currently popular term, graft-versus host (GVH) reaction, is not used here. Whether this reaction is proceeding in a host, who by means of radiation or other immunosuppressive therapy, is made tolerant to a thrifty hematopoietic tissue graft from a genetically unrelated donor, or the reaction is proceeding in a nonirradiated, nonthymectomized, but immunologically immature host who harbours a thrifty hematopoietic tissue graft from an almost genetically similar, older hybrid donor, the following are characteristic of the GVH reaction: [23]

1. Failure of many organs to grow or develop normally.

2. Increased susceptibility to infection.

3. Atrophy or absence of small lymphocytes throughout the lymphoid organs.

4. Enlargement of some lymphoid organs, particularly the spleen, owing to hyperplasia of large pyroninophilic cells resembling plasmablasts or large lymphocytes. Since all but the last can be found in many nongrafted neonatally thymectomized animals, heavily irradiated young animals, and young animals given massive doses of cortisol, it must be presumed that hyperplasia of large pyroninophilic cells is somehow related to the graft, to some form of antigenic stimulation, or to both.

Some assume that the hyperplastic, large pyroninophilic cells are more or less purely of graft origin (i.e. grafted lymphocytes which have circulated, colonized, dedifferentiated, and transformed) and that they are producing antibodies and/or lymphocytes which react against the host to produce the wasting or runt disease manifest.[23] This point of view is supported by the following findings.

1. Isotope label, such as [3]HT, from labeled donor lymphocytes appears in significant concentration in the large pyroninophilic cells in the lymphoid organs of the host.[70]

2. Karyotype label, such as Y chromosome, from donor lymphocytes characteristically carrying this label can be found in mitotically dividing pyroninophilic cells in the lymphoid organs of the immunologically tolerant host.[280]

3. Lymphocytes, under some circumstances, can destroy other cells.

It is possible, however, that the large pyroninophilic cells are actually host cells which are relatively insensitive to radiation or other forms of immunosuppressive therapy and which continue to differentiate from the reticular cells *in situ*, grow, and react toward the continued influx of foreign antigens. This occurs because the

→

From a geomedical point of view, it is important to look upon the small lymphocytes and their DNA not only as endogenous agents which feed, protect, and destroy other cells but also as agents which are extremely sensitive to exogenous agents, such as radioactive isotopes and mustard gases originally intended for use in warfare. As we learn more about the biologic effects of these agents, about similar agents continually being developed for bellicose and clinical usage, and about the potent chemicals

---

relatively radiosensitive, chemically suppressed, or otherwise undeveloped small lymphocytes are incapable of destroying the cellular source of these foreign antigens. This point of view is supported by the following considerations:

1. A significant concentration of isotope label, such as [3]HT, in the large pyroninophilic cells can be explained simply by the donation of DNA or its label from labeled donor lymphocytes, whether the host is immunologically competent or not. Moreover, a significant concentration of isotope label in other types of cells, such as intestinal crypt cells, regenerating hepatic polygonal cells, and regenerating fibroblasts, cannot be readily explained on the basis of donor lymphocyte transformation into such unrelated cell types (see Chap. 16, F-H).

2. As long as the host remains tolerant to foreign DNA (see Chap. 16, B), the finding of karyotype label, such as Y-chromosome, in large dividing pyroninophilic cells [293] can be explained simply by donation coupled with temporary expression of donor lymphocyte codes in recipient cells, normally accustomed to reutilizing DNA from small lymphocytes (see Chap. 16, E). Further experiments related to the transfer factor obtained by Lawrence from lymphocyte extracts may help to substantiate this consideration (see Chap. 16, H).

3. In healthy individuals, as well as in immunologically suppressed ones, hyperplasia of large pyroninophilic cells in regional lymphoid organs usually indicates reaction of host cells toward antigens emanating from a graft or from bacteria (see Chap. 18, B). As the spleen appears particularly active in processing antigens which reach the arteriovenous circulation and therefore can be expected to process a relatively large share of the circulating antigenic output of the bone marrow, it should not be surprising to find a prominent reaction there when bone marrow is transplanted successfully between individuals.

4. Whether or not hyperplasia of large pyroninophilic cells is manifest, absence or atrophy of small lymphocytes throughout the lymphoid organs is commonly associated with wasting and increased susceptibility to infections, especially in young free-living animals.[23]

Pursuant to such considerations, the term, graft-versus-host reaction is not used in the same sense as the growth failure, wasting, wasting disease, lack of thrift, runt disease, or secondary disease which accompanies experimental or therapeutic immunosuppression, whether or not a graft has been applied. As sensitization appears to be a prerequisite to reactivity on the part of lymphocytes, it is doubtful that unselected transfused lymphocytes actually react specifically toward host cells. It is not inconceivable, however, that the "immunosuppressed" host can mount abortive reactions toward antigens emanating from any kind of transfused cells.

with which we are polluting our air, our fields, and our streams, it is our responsibility as physicians to advise our duly elected representatives, lest these statesmen unwittingly fail to control the dissemination of pollutants at home [267] or, in conjunction with their responsible counterparts abroad, unwittingly turn loose a quantity of radioactive materials [268] sufficient to reduce the human race and all forms of life containing DNA (and the environment in which all are feeding and breathing) into forms of substrate which cannot be utilized for purposeful growth by any one or any living thing for an indeterminate period of time.

Chapter 20

AND BACK TO THE GUT

S O FAR WE HAVE considered that molecules newly absorbed via the intestinal mucosa are transformed by intestinal lymphoid tissue into lymph; that this lymph flows centrally into the arteriovenous system to carry nourishment to outlying lymphoid and nonlymphoid tissues; that lymphoid and nonlymphoid tissues mutually exchange information via the peripheral lymph which comes from the tissues and the central lymph which flows from the lymphoid organs into the arteriovenous circulation; and that energy exchanges are involved during this complex transfer of substrate and information. It is pertinent, therefore, to think about what happens to the share of substrate, information, and energy which returns to the gut via the circulating plasma and small lymphocytes. While the answers may be speculative, an approach to the question can be made by discussing the plasma and lymphocytes which return to the gut in terms of decrements.

Irrespective of the precise cellular or tissue sites of origin, the plasma and small lymphocytes brought in via the intestinal arterioles may pass onward or be reutilized in the following decremental order:

1. Most will pass onward into the mesenteric veins to be reutilized in the liver and later in remaining organs in the body.

2. Some may pass into the interstices and be reutilized there for growth and function in cells mostly lymphoid.

3. Some may pass onward into the intestinal mucosal cells and be reutilized there for growth and function.

4. Some may pass or migrate all the way through into the intestinal lumen to be further disposed of there.

Out of the first decrement, the intestinal reutilization of larger plasma molecules and small lymphocytes need not be taken into account for they will have passed through the capillary bed of the intestine and are on their way to the liver. It is necessary to consider primarily the small molecules such as oxygen, water, salts, glucose, and amino acids, which diffuse relatively rapidly from the arterioles to be reutilized in the gut, and other small molecules such as carbon dioxide, water, simple sugars, amino acids, and short-chain fatty acids, which diffuse relatively rapidly from the gut into the intestinal arteriovenous capillaries.

Out of the second decrement, reutilization of relatively large slow-diffusing molecules and rapidly emigrating small lymphocytes is an important factor to be taken into account. For, within the interstitial lymphoid tissue of the intestine, they may be reutilized for growth and the subsequent production of lymph. As already mentioned (see Chap. 15), if the extraintestinal supply of lymphocytes (or their disintegration products) is cut off, as occurs after neonatal thymectomy, the intestinal lymphoid tissue remains relatively atrophic, growth rate in remaining lymphoid and nonlymphoid tissues is retarded, and the thymectomized animal usually ceases to thrive in the ambient environment.

Out of the third decrement, reutilization of slow-moving large plasma molecules and fast-migrating small lymphocytes within the intestinal mucosal cells (see Figs. 28 and 29) undoubtedly plays an essential role in their growth. Moreover, as mentioned on page 142, reutilization of the information and energy carried in the DNA of small lymphocytes may play an important role in directing their subsequent function.

Out of the fourth decrement, there are at least three possible pathways of disposition of the plasma constituents and lymphocytes which have, respectively, diffused or migrated actively from the arterioles all the way through into the lumen of the gut. The possible pathways include the following, singly or in combination:

1. Digestion within the lumen of the gut, a pathway which will allow the digested products of exuding plasma and intraluminal lymphocytes to be selectively reabsorbed, or excreted as small molecules.

2. Fecal excretion, a pathway which will allow the body to get rid of plasma constituents, lymphocytes, or their breakdown

104. Perry, S., Craddock, C. G., Ventzke, L., Crepaldi, G., and Lawrence, J. S.: Rate of production of P^{32}-labeled lymphocytes. *Blood, 14*:50–59, 1959.

105. Cronkite, E. P., Jansen, C. R., Cottier, H., Kanti, R., and Sipe, C. R.: Lymphocyte production measured by extracorporeal irradiation, cannulation, and labeling techniques. *Ann N Y Acad Sci, 113*:566–577, 1964.

106. Little, J. R., Brecher, G., Bradley, T. R., and Rose, S.: Determination of lymphocyte turnover by continuous infusion of H^3-thymidine. *Blood, 19*:236–242, 1962.

107. Robinson, S. H., Brecher, G., Lourie, I. S., and Haley, J. E.: Leucocyte labeling in rats during and after continuous infusion of tritiated thymidine. Implications for lymphocyte longevity and DNA re-utilization. *Blood, 26*:281–295, 1965.

108. Leblond, C. P. and Walker, B. E.: Renewal of cell populations. *Physiol Rev, 36*:255–276, 1956.

109. Leblond, C. P. and Messier, B.: Renewal of chief cells and goblet cells in the small intestine as shown by radioautography after injection of thymidine-H^3 into mice. *Anat Rec, 132*:247–259, 1959.

110a. Leblond, C. P.: Classification of cell populations on the basis of their proliferative behavior. In *NCI Monograph 14, International Symposium on the Control of Cell Division and the Induction of Cancer.* Washington, U.S. Government Printing Office, 1966, pp. 119–150.

110b. Messier, B. and Leblond, C. P.: Cell proliferation and migration as revealed by autoradiography after injection of thymidine-H^3 into male rats and mice. *Amer J Anat, 106*:247–285, 1960.

111. Cronkite, E. P., Fliedner, T. M., Bond, V. P., Rubini, J. R., Brecher, G., and Quastler, H.: Dynamics of hemopoietic proliferation in man and mice studied by H^3-thymidine incorporation into DNA. *Ann N Y Acad Sci, 77*:803–820, 1959.

112. Craddock, C. G.: Production and distribution of granulocytes and the control of granulocyte release. In Wolstenholme, G. E. W. and O'Connor, M. (Eds.): *Haemopoiesis—Cell Production and Its Regulation.* Boston, Little, Brown, 1961, pp. 237–261.

113. Andreason, E. and Ottesen, J.: Significance of the various lymphoid organs in the lymphocyte production in the albino rat. *Acta Path Microbiol Scand,* suppl. *54*:25–32, 1944.

114. Andreason, E. and Ottesen, J.: Studies on the lymphocyte production. Investigations on the nucleic acid turnover in the lymphoid organs. *Acta Physiol Scand, 10*:258–270, 1945.

115. Yoffey, J. M., Hanks, G. A., and Kelly, L.: Some problems of lymphocyte production. *Ann N Y Acad Sci, 73*:47–78, 1958.

116. Osgood, E. E., Tivey, H., Davidson, K. B., Seaman, A. J., and Li, J. G.: The relative rates of formation of new leukocytes in patients with acute and chronic leukemias: measured by the uptake of radioactive phosphorous in the isolated desoxyribose nucleic acid. *Cancer, 5*:331–335, March 1952.

117. Everett, N. B., Rieke, W. O., and Caffrey, R. W.: The kinetics of small lymphocytes in the rat, with special reference to those of thymic origin. In Good, R. A. and Gabrielson, A. E. (Eds.): *The Thymus in Immunobiology.* New York, Hoeber, 1964, pp. 291–297.

118. Trowell, O. A.: Reutilization of lymphocytes in lymphopoiesis. *J Biophys Cytol, 3*:317–318, 1957.

119. Hamilton, L. D.: Control and function of the lymphocyte. *Ann N Y Acad Sci, 73*:39–46, 1958.

120. Yoffey, J. M. (Ed.): *The Lymphocyte in Immunology and Haemopoiesis.* (Bristol Lymphocyte Symposium, April 1966.) London, Edward Arnold, Ltd., 1966.

121. Leblond, C. P. and Sainte-Marie, G.: Thymus-cell population dynamics. In Good, R. A. and Gabrielson, A. E. (Eds.): *The Thymus in Immunobiology.* New York, Hoeber, 1964, pp. 207–226.

122. Everett, N. B. and Tyler, R. W.: Radioautographic studies of the reticular and lymphoid cells in germinal centers of lymph nodes. In Cottier, H. *et al.* (Eds.): *Germinal Centers in Immune Responses.* New York, Springer-Verlag, 1967, pp. 145–151.

123. Moore, M. A. S. and Owen, J. J. T.: Hypothesis: Stem cell migration in developing myeloid and lymphoid systems. *Lancet,* Sept. 23, 1967, pp. 658–659.

124. Roitt, I. M., Greaves, M. F., Torrigiani, G., Brostoff, J., and Playfair, J. H. L.: The cellular basis of immunologic responses. *Lancet,* Aug. 16, 1969, pp. 267–370.

125. Jordan, H. E.: Comparative hematology. In Downey, H. (Ed.): *Handbook of Hematology.* New York, Hoeber, 1938, vol. 2, pp. 699–862.

126. Gilmour, J. R.: Normal haemopoiesis in intrauterine and neonatal life. *J Path Bact, 52*:25–55, 1941.

127. Trowell, O. A.: The lymphocyte. *Int Rev Cytol, 7*:235–293, 1958.

128. Drinker, C. K. and Yoffey, J. M.: *Lymphatics, Lymph and Lymphoid Tissue.* Cambridge, Harvard University Press, 1941.

129. Hofmeister, F.: Untersuchungen Über Resorption und Assimilation der Nährstoffe. *Arch Exp Path Pharmkol, 19*:1–83, 1885.

130. Ivy, A. C.: Gastrointestinal changes in the rat on realimentation. *Amer J Physiol, 195*:216–220, 1958.

131. MacKenzie, D. W., Whipple, A. O., and Wintersteiner, M. P.: Studies on microscopic anatomy and physiology of living transilluminated mammalian spleens. *Amer J Anat, 68*:397–456, 1941.

132. White, A. and Dougherty, T. F.: The role of lymphocytes in normal and immune globulin production and the mode of release of globulin from lymphocytes. *Ann N Y Acad Sci, 46*:859–882, 1942.

133. White, A.: Influence of endocrine secretions on the structure and function of lymphoid tissue. In *Harvey Lectures*. Springfield, Thomas, 1950, pp. 43–70.

134. Beguin. Quoted in Andrew, W., and Sosa, J. M.: Mitotic division and degeneration of lymphocytes within cells of intestinal epithelium in young and in adult white mice. *Anat Rec, 97*:63–97, 1947.

135. Andrew, W. and Sosa, J. M.: Mitotic division and degeneration of lymphocytes within cells of intestinal epithelium in young and in adult white mice. *Anat Rec, 97*:63–97, 1947.

136. Andrew, W.: Lymphocyte transformation in epithelium. *J Nat Cancer Inst, 35*:113–137, 1965.

137. Darlington, D. and Rogers, A. W.: Epithelial lymphocytes in the small intestine of the mouse. *J Anat, 100*:813–830, 1966.

138. Meader, R. D. and Landers, D. F.: Electron and light microscopic observations on relationships between lymphocytes and intestinal epithelium. *Amer J Anat, 121*:763–773, 1967.

139. Fichtelius, K. E., Yunis, E. J., and Good, R. A.: Occurrence of lymphocytes within the gut epithelium of normal and neonatally thymectomized mice. *Proc Soc Exp Biol Med, 128*:185–188, 1968.

140. Fichtelius, K. E.: The gut epithelium—a first level lymphoid organ? *Exp Cell Res, 49*:87–104, 1968.

141. Kindred, J. E.: A quantitative study of the haemopoietic organs of young albino rats. *Amer J Anat, 67*:99–149, 1940.

142. Kindred, J. E.: A quantitative study of the haemopoietic organs of young adult albino rats. *Amer J Anat, 71*:207–243, 1942.

143. Ebert, R. H., Sanders, A. G., and Florey, H. W.: Observations on lymphocytes in chambers in the rabbit's ears. *Brit J Exp Path, 21*:212–218, Aug, 1940.

144. Sherwin, R. P.: *The Embattled Cell.* A movie sponsored by the American Cancer Society, 1967.

145. Shields, J. W.: An evaluation of splenic puncture as a procedure in the diagnosis of hematologic disorders. Mayo Foundation Thesis, Jan. 1956.

146. Shields, J. W. and Hargraves, M. M.: An evaluation of splenic puncture. *Proc Staff Meeting, Mayo Clinic, 31*:440–453, 1956.

147. Downey, H. and Weidenreich, F.: Ueber die Bildung der Lymphocyten in Lymphdruesen und Milz. *Arch Anat Entwicklungsgesch, 80*:306, 1912.

148. Sabin, F. R.: Bone marrow. In Cowdry, E. V. (Ed.): *Special Cytology.* New York, Hoeber, 1932, pp. 507–527.

149. Sabin, F. R.: Bone marrow. *Physiol Rev, 8*:191–244, April, 1928.

150. Shields, J. W.: On the relationship between growing blood cells and blood vessels. *Acta Haematol, 24*:319–329, 1960.

151. Fliedner, T. M.: On the origin of tingible bodies in germinal centers. In Cottier, H. *et al.* (Eds.): *Germinal Centers in Immune Responses.* New York, Springer-Verlag, 1967, pp. 218–221.

152. Brachet, J.: The localization and the role of ribonucleic acid in the cell. *Ann N Y Acad Sci, 50*:861–869, 1950.

153. Michels, N. A.: The plasma cell: A critical review of its morphogenesis, function and developmental capacity under normal and under abnormal conditions. *Arch Path, 11*:775–793, 1931.

154. Weidenreich, F.: Das Gefaess-System der menschlichen Milz. *Arch Mikr Anat, 58*:247–376, 1901.

155. Jaeger, E.: Die Gefaessversorgung der Malpighischen Koerperchen in der Milz. *Z. Zellforsch, 8*:578–601, 1929.

156. Maximow, A.: Bindegewebe und blutbildende Gewebe. In Moellendorf, V. (Ed.): *Handbuch d mikr Anat des Menschen.* Berlin, Springer, 1927 (2,pt.1) p. 23.

157. Knisely, M. H.: Microscopic observations of the circulatory system of living unstimulated mammalian spleens. *Anat Rec, 65*:23–50, 1936.

158. Ehrich, W. E.: The role of the lymphocytes in the circulation of lymph. *Ann N Y Acad Sci, 46*:823–857, 1946.

159. Whipple, A. O., Parpart, A. K., and Chang, J. J.: A study of the circulation of the blood in the spleen of the living mouse. *Ann Surg, 140*:266–269, 1954.

160. Krogh, A.: *The Anatomy and Physiology of Capillaries.* New Haven, Yale University Press, 1929.

161. Zweifach, B. W.: The character and distribution of the blood capillaries. *Anat Rec, 73*:475–495, 1939.

162. Brånemark, I.: Experimental investigation of microcirculation in bone marrow. *Angiology, 12*:293–305, 1961.

163. Shields, J. W.: Personal observation.

164. Smith, C.: The microscopic anatomy of the thymus. In Good, R. A. and Gabrielson, A. E. (Eds.): *The Thymus in Immunology.* New York, Hoeber, pp. 71–84.

165. Kostowiecki, M.: Development and degeneration of the second type of Hassall's corpuscles in the thymus of the guinea pig. *Anat Rec, 142*:195–203, Feb 1962.

166. Whipple, G. H.: *The Dynamic Equilibrium of Body Proteins.* Springfield, Thomas, 1956.

167. Mannik, M. and Kunkel, W. G.: The immunoglobulins. In Samter, M. and Alexander, H. L. (Eds.): *Immunological Diseases,* Boston, Little, Brown, 1965, pp. 278–304.

Section 3

ON THE INTRAVASCULAR SECRETION OF
BLOOD AND LYMPH

Chapter 23

INTRODUCTION

JUST AS THE BLOOD cells would be stranded, unable to flow anywhere and therefore useless, were it not for the plasma, so would whole blood (plasma and cells) be stranded, unable to flow in a purposeful direction, and therefore useless, were it not for the vessels. With such basic considerations in mind, it is my purpose here to review and analyze the development of the blood, lymph, and vessels as they relate to one another, and as all relate to the nutrition of remaining tissues in the body.

This analysis is necessary for at least two reasons. First, although it is well known that the whole blood, the blood-forming organs, and the vessels all take their embryologic origin from mesenchyme and that the blood cells continue to take their origin in the perivascular reticulum (reticular connective tissue) of the adult hematopoietic organs,[1] it remains to be elucidated how, during adult life, blood elements, particularly those lacking the power of independent motility, i.e. erythrocytes, thrombocytes, and free extracellular proteins, gain access to and egress from the vascular system—a system still considered by many to be a closed one lined entirely by endothelium. Second, although it is known that the plasma and blood cells develop simultaneously from mesenchyme long before the liver is embryologically demarcated, it is assumed currently on the basis of certain isotope experiments [3-5] that the bulk of the plasma proteins are secreted by the entodermal (parenchymal) cells of the liver. This is an assumption open to serious challenge on the basis of phylogenetic, ontogenetic, osmotic, and functional grounds.[6]

The key to these problems will be found through analysis of the manner in which plasma develops, how it flows, and the make-up of the colloid osmotic pressure which it contains. Therefore, the analysis will proceed with particular emphasis on the movements of water, other small molecules, and patterns of blood and lymph flow which serve as important determinants of differentiations involved.

Chapter 24

AN ANALYSIS OF EMBRYOLOGIC DEVELOPMENT

A. THE GENERAL SEQUENCE OF DEVELOPMENT

PHYLOGENETICALLY and embryologically, the development of the vascular system lags behind the development of the connective tissue and the blood. In the lower orders of multicellular organisms such as the sponges and the coelenterates, where the distance between internal cells remotely located from the food supply is sufficiently small to allow for adequate nutrition by diffusion from cells located close to the environmental food supply, only mesoblastic connective tissue separates the cell layers and serves as the sole pathway for intercellular nutritional exchange.[7] Facilitating the dissemination of nutrients in more complicated organisms such as flatworms, one finds free fluid vaguely resembling blood [8] percolating through spaces or lacunae within the mesoblastic or mesenchymal connective tissue which separates the ectoderm and entoderm.[7] These lacunae are lined by this connective tissue, not by specific endothelium.[9] Ascending the phylogenetic scale from the nemerteans through the vertebrates, there is increasing specialization of the middle or mesodermal germ layer to expedite the transport of oxygen and nutrients to the bulkier, more widely separated, and more specialized mass of tissues which arise out of all three primary germ layers. To facilitate the dissemination of nutrients in the latter group of organisms the blood, the chambers of the heart, a system of ducts lined by specific endothelium, and a separate lymphatic apparatus develop in this order from the mesenchyme (which is the counterpart of the mesoblast in these higher forms of phylogenetic development).

315

B. VERTEBRATE MESENCHYME DEVELOPMENT

In vertebrate embryos, this developmental sequence is recapitulated during the growth and differentiation of the mesenchymal connective tissue. This jelly-like tissue makes its first appearance by differentiation from cells located at the blastopore lip [10] and from the somite mesoderm.[14] It grows then as a syncytium which spreads the ectoderm and entoderm apart.[10-13] Initially, this mesenchyme constitutes the matrix through which all nutritive exchange takes place between the separate cell layers. Later, as the embryo increases in bulk, the mesenchyme commences to give rise to the first blood in close spatial relationship to the nutrient-laden yolk sac entoderm.[10-14] Here, the blood plasma arises through dissolution of expanding local mesenchyme, while the blood cells arise simultaneously through "rounding up" and separation of primitive free cells (principally nucleated erythrocytes) from the hypertrophic mesenchymal syncytium.[10-15] Separate puddles of whole blood, thus formed from plasma and cells, then commence to coalesce.[10-13] By the progressive coalescence of many separate puddles, there is demarcated a blood-filled lucanar system contained in the mesenchymal syncytium which immediately underlies and supports the yolk sac entoderm.[10-13] It is particularly significant to note that as time and growth progress, more blood filled lacunae arise out of the mesenchymal syncytium and coalesce in a progression which proceeds from the yolk sac into body areas successively more remote from the yolk sac.[10-13]

When a blood-filled lacunar system, formed by the centripetal fusion of many separate puddles, has invaded the body area destined to become the anterior mediastinum, the heart muscle develops from the local mesoderm and commences to impel the centrifugal flow of the blood within the system.[10-13] After the heart has developed sufficiently to constitute an effective pump, those segments of the previously established lacunar system which carry a constant flow of blood away from the heart become recognizable as arteries, while those segments which carry a constant flow of blood toward the heart become recognizable as veins.[10] As these particular segments of the previously demarcated lacunar system become transformed into definitive vessels, the mesenchymal syncytium directly lining individual lacunae progressively flattens and differentiates into endothelial cells.[9,16] At the same time, hematopoiesis ceases locally.[16] The definitive vessels outlined by this transformation then continue their growth by reproduction of endothelial cells and by the addition of muscular coats.[10,17] Meanwhile, as the definitive vessels are demarcated in this manner throughout the general body mesenchyme, hematopoiesis shifts to special hematopoietic organs [14,18] having characteristic patterns of cellular differentiation and characteristic patterns of blood and lymph flow (see below).

C. ANALYSIS OF EMBRYONAL HEMOPOIESIS AND VASCULOGENESIS IN RELATION TO THE MOVEMENT OF MOLECULAR SUBSTRATE

As pointed out by Bloom [1] hematopoiesis in embryonic and postnatal animals is one of the most controversial subjects in histology. Controversial, also, remain many aspects of vasculogenesis.[19-23] It is pertinent, therefore, to analyze certain features of hemopoiesis and vasculogenesis which are interrelated, focusing particular attention during the analysis on the potential sources of molecular substrate necessary for mesenchymal growth and differentiation into blood, lymph, and vessels.

1. The Spatial and Temporal Sequence of Development

According to the embryologic descriptions,[10-14] the circulatory system takes its early origin not as a vascular tree springing out from the heart but as a disorganized system of separate blood-filled lacunae which arise out of expanding, differentiating mesenchyme in a sequence paralleling the pathway of molecular diffusion from the yolk sac entoderm into the body of the embryo. The entire body mesenchyme is initially hematopoietic,[10-15,24] forming blood from molecular substrate which can only reach each successive area of the body through diffusion* within the

---

* Thermal and atomic energy impel all molecules to move by diffusion through air, water, sols, gels, cells, tissues, and solids at velocities which are proportional to molecular solubility and inversely proportional to molecular weight.

gelatinous mesenchyme, since there is no other established pathway through which the molecular substrate necessary for extended
tissue growth can move. The blood-filled lucanae which arise
out of this mesenchyme initially are lined with the same mesenchyme out of which the plasma and free blood cells arise.[10-15] It
is only later, after many blood-filled lacunae have coalesced,
the heart has developed, and the circulation has commenced,
that some components of the mesenchyme flatten, demarcate from
the mesenchymal syncytium, and become recognizable as common
vascular endothelial cells identical with those of adult
vessels.[9,15,16] This final transformation from a blood-filled connective tissue lacuna into a definitive vessel lined by endothelium
occurs after the advent of blood flow,[16] and along the lines of
flow which become progressively established from and to the
heart.[10] This direction is different from the one in which the
anlage of the circulatory system was originally established. It
appears, therefore, that vasculogenesis involves two spatially and
temporally related processes:

1. The successive centripetal formation of whole blood as a
result of utilization of diffusing molecules for mesenchymal hypertrophy and differentiation.

2. The successive centrifugal differentiation, with the establishment of blood flow, of this same mesenchymal tissue into
endothelial tubes to surround the previously formed blood.

2. Formation of Whole Blood from the Mesenchyme

According to the classic embryologic descriptions,[11-14] the blood
is noted to arise in each body area in the form of whole blood.
This point requires more emphasis. Although the blood cells are
the microscopically prominent entities taking origin from the
hypertrophic mesenchyme of each body area, the blood plasma
is noted to arise simultaneously by dissolution of (gelatinous)
mesenchyme [10-13] and by cytoplasmic secretion from components
within the mesenchyme.[15] Without this plasma, the blood could
not flow. Without the proteins (colloids) in this plasma, the
blood could not osmotically retain its water within the vessels once

sufficient hydrostatic pressure is generated by the heart to impel active flow.

It is significant to note in this connection that the blood cells and blood plasma are formed as described before the liver is embryologically demarcated and before the placenta is demarcated in mammals.[10] It would be impossible, therefore, for the liver or the placenta to be the source of the plasma or its proteins during this early prehepatic and preplacental period of embryogenesis. Moreover, in oviparous species, neither the mother nor the placenta is the immediate source of the embryo's circulating plasma or its constituent proteins.

3. The Involution of Hematopoiesis in Relation to the Systemic Vessels and its Evolution in Special Hematopoietic Organs Containing Sinusoids

The establishment of the definitive vessels containing flowing blood in the yolk sac and in the general body mesenchyme signals the disappearance of blood formation as it pertains to these particular vessels. The continued process of blood formation, then, becomes relegated to the mesenchymal component of the liver (temporarily), the spleen, the lymphatic organs, and the bone marrow, where hematopoiesis flourishes, in each instance, in close relation to special circulatory channels known as sinusoids.

a. The Liver

The first special blood-forming organ to appear after the establishment of the circulation is in the mesenchymal portion of the liver.[10,14,18] Here, about the vessels which carry the nutrient-laden blood from the yolk sac and later from the placenta, the perivascular mesenchyme undergoes hypertrophy and differentiates.[25] As a result of this hypertrophy and differentiation, more plasma and more blood cells arise.[25] The separate puddles of blood thus formed from plasma and cells coalesce, one with the next.[25] At the same time, these puddles establish connections with the capillary vessels similarily but previously demarcated during the yolk sac period of hemopoiesis.[25] Many of the newly formed perivascular blood puddles eventually connect with the previously established vessels and change into vascular thoroughfares like those in the general body mesenchyme.[26] However, many puddles continue in a situation where connections with the definitive vessels are only intermittently patent. During adult life, this situation is illustrated during transillumination of living liver tissue where it is observed that flow from the established arteries to the established veins is intermittent in certain channels.[26] These intermittently patent channels, lined by reticuloendothelium, become recognized as the hepatic venous sinusoids of adult life.[26,27]

For a period of time, the hepatic mesenchyme constitutes the principal blood-forming organ of the embryo.[10,18] However, as an arteriovenous oxygen difference becomes appreciable [28] and the vascular system develops further, hemopoiesis subsides in the liver and commences in definitive lymphoid and myeloid organs.[10,14,18]

b. The Lymphatic Apparatus

The development of the lymphatic apparatus is identical with that in the anlage of the cardiovascular system, but the direction of development is reversed, being centrifugal rather than centripetal.[10,19-23] Whereas the anlage of the cardiovascular system develops along the pathway of molecular diffusion from the yolk sac entoderm toward the body area in which the heart will develop, the lymphatic system develops along the pathway of outward diffusion of molecules from arterioles after the heart has developed and has commenced to impel the circulation of blood. The developmental sequence commences in the neck adjacent to the outflow tracts of the heart, continues along the course of tiny arteries which will become thoracic and abdominal aorta, and is completed in close proximity to the developing arterioles of the periphery.[20-23] Following the progressive demarcation of definitive arterioles in each of these body areas, the local periarteriolar mesenchyme progressively undergoes hypertrophy and differentiation which results in the formation of lymphatics and lymph nodes.[20-23,29-31]

The lymphatics are demarcated when the local periarteriolar

mesenchyme undergoes sufficient hypertrophy and differentiation to form lymphocytes and lymph plasma.[20-23,29-31] Some components of the local mesenchymal syncytium "round up" to form lymphocytes, while others dissolve to create lymph plasma.[20-23,29-31] As portions of the syncytium dissolve, some of the lymphocytes are set free to migrate within the newly formed lymph plasma.[20-23,29-31] Arising thus out of the periarteolar mesenchyme are puddles of whole lymph. By the repetitive centrifugal coalescence of isolated lymph puddles, there is established a lymph-filled lacunar system completely separate from the arterial system and separate from the venous system, except for tributary connections to a few tiny blood-filled channels which later will become the great veins of the neck.[10,20-23] These tributary connections become recognized as the thoracic and cervical lymph ducts.[10,20-23]

Certain segments of this separate lacunar system eventually become thoroughfares for the rapid circulation of lymph.[10,20-23] Here, the inner components of the mesenchymal syncytium flatten, become separate from the syncytium, and develop into common vascular endothelial cells, similar to those of the established arteries and veins.[9,20-23,31] Still later, muscular coats are added, so that these particular segments of the lymphatic apparatus come to resemble smaller arteries or veins.[9,10] It is noteworthy, however, that the lymphatic thoroughfares never achieve the highly organized structure of arteries or veins.[1] At the same time, it should be pointed out that the daily volume of lymph flow, even in animals possessing lymph hearts,* remains far below the daily volume of arteriovenous blood flow.[32]

As the lymphatic thoroughfares are being demarcated, some of the mesenchymal connective tissue along these demarcating thoroughfares undergoes a relatively intense hypertrophy which results in the development of lymph nodes.[20-23,29-31] The nodes develop in such a manner that thoroughfares are always interupted somewhere along their course by nodal tissue.[32] Where

---

* In the majority of vertebrates, lymph flow is induced by skeletal muscular contractions and by pulsations from adjacent blood vessels.[32]

the nodes will develop, their development is signaled by a relatively intense concentration of recognizable arterioles.[28-31,33] Surrounding these arterioles, the mesenchyme undergoes intensive hypertrophy, undergoes hyperplasia, and then differentiates into reticulum (a protoplasmic syncytium traversed by a network of fine fibrils) densely packed with developing lymphocytes.[29-31,33] While this lymphocyte-packed reticulum forms a dense sheath around the arterioles, it continues simultaneously as the integral lining of lymph spaces which are located in the center and at the periphery of the nodular masses of lymphocytes which continue to develop from and within the reticulum.[29,31] These lymph spaces in the nodes lined by the reticulum are called the central and peripheral sinusoids, respectively.[1,34] The flattened reticulum lining the sinusoids is classified with the reticuloendothelium[35,36] to be described subsequently. By the repetetive establishment of connections through coalescence between the peripheral sinusoids and the lymphatic thoroughfares outside of the nodes, the links in lymphatic chain are forged.[20-23,29-31]

Within the central portions of the nodes, the establishment of connections becomes so complicated as a result of the nodular hypertrophy of adjacent lymphoid tissue that the central sinusoidal system take on the character of mazes.[29,31] Through these mazes, the peripheral to central movement of lymph is best described by the term "percolation" rather than "flow."

c. The Spleen

The development of the spleen is similar to that of the lymph nodes in that following the outward pathway of molecular diffusion from developing, intensely concentrated arterioles, the mesenchyme of the splenic rudiment undergoes hypertrophy and differentiation into reticulum densely packed with developing lymphocytes.[29-30,33] The latter continue to proliferate in that portion of the reticulum which remains closely apposed to and "sheathes" the arterioles.[29-30,33] As a result of this hypertrophy and differential growth, the splenic rudiment enlarges rapidly and becomes displaced through growth into the peritoneal cavity.[10,29,23] Meanwhile, within the enlarging splenic rudiment, the differentiation of erythrocytes continues within that portion of the reticulum which surrounds circulatory channels wherein flow remains less constant than in the arterioles or in arteriovenous thoroughfares.[10,29-30,33] These circulatory channels in which flow remains inconstant [45,46] becomes recognized as the (portal) venous sinusoids of the spleen,[1,10,14,33,35-36] and the flattened reticulum [29-31] which lines them becomes recognized as reticuloendothelium.[29-36] Still later (in mammals), when the heart transforms from a three-chambered into a four-chambered pump and the arteriovenous oxygen difference approaches that of the newborn, erythrocytopoiesis subsides in the spleen.[10,28] The spleen then becomes a predominantly lymphoid organ which differs from the lymph nodes primarily in the fact that hemopoietic activity continues in a relationship with (portal) venous sinusoids, instead of in a relationship with lymphatic sinusoids.[32]

d. The Bone Marrow

The development of the bone marrow is similar to that of the lymph nodes and spleen in that following the pathway of molecular diffusion around developing blood vessels, the mesenchyme of each marrow rudiment undergoes hypertrophy and differentiation.[10,14] As each marrow rudiment enlarges as a result of this hypertrophy and differentiation, it grows into an adjacent cartilage.[10,14] While the invasion of cartilage is proceeding, each marrow rudiment begins to show a pattern of differential growth which is different from that of the lymph nodes in that lymphatics are not developed inside of the cartilage [32]; and which differs from that of the lymph nodes and the spleen in that arterioles do not become intensively concentrated.* Instead, the bulk of perivascular mesenchymal hypertrophy and differentiation results in the continued formation of erythrocytes, megakaryocytes, and granulocytes within the reticulum [1,14,36] which surrounds irregularly shaped circulatory channels having a slow, intermit-

---

* It is pertinent to note that arterioles are relatively few and far between in the bone marrow [28] and that veins remain to be demonstrated in the follicular and medullary reticulum of lymphoid tissue.[39] These local variations in vascular pattern seem to supply optimal local conditions for differentiated blood cell growth insofar as oxygen tension, pH, and carbon dioxide tension are concerned.[28]

tent circulation.[37,38]* These channels, recognized as venous sinusoids, are lined by reticuloendothelium.[35,36]

4. Summary and Conclusions

In this part of the analysis, the data from the literature are organized to suggest that:

1. Embryonal hematopoiesis and vasculogenesis take place as a result of two sequential processes:

a. The preliminary mesenchymal utilization of diffusing molecular substrate first from the yolk sac entoderm and later from demarcating vessels in order to form isolated accumulations of whole blood or lymph by means of hypertrophy, differentiation, and dissolution.

b. The subsequent differentiation of the local mesenchyme in each body area into endothelial tubes to encase the newly formed blood or lymph when flow actually commences as a result of fusion of separate blood or lymph accumulations under the impetus supplied by rhythmic cardiac or skeletal muscular contractions.

2. The blood or lymph, as each arises from the mesenchyme, is created in the form of whole blood or whole lymph so that flow and the colloid osmotic retention of plasma water are assured before flow actually commences.

3. As each definitive hematopoietic organ arises from the mesenchyme, it develops in relation to venous or lymphathic sinusoids wherein flow remains inconstant.

4. Each definitive hematopoietic organ also develops in a relation to arteries, veins, and lymphatics, which is specific and quantitatively different in each organ (see Fig. 1b). These quantitative differences allow not only for a distinctive type of vascular drainage from each organ but also for a perivascular tissue environment with optimal oxygen tension, carbon dioxide

---

* While it is agreed that the granulocytes and megakaryocytes take their respective origins in extravascular mesenchymal tissue, it was never settled whether the first generation of erythroblasts (megaloblasts) arise from endothelial cells [11-13, 37, 38] or directly from mesenchyme.[14] The controversy possibly revolves about what is to be defined as an endothelial cell, e.g. any cell syncytially arranged or isolated, phagocytic or nonphagocytic, and lining a space containing blood or lymph; or a single nonphagocytic cell with definite stainable margins forming the lining of a tubular vessel.

tension, and pH for the extended growth of differentiated cell types in each organ.

D. ANALYSIS OF VASCULAR DIFFERENTIATION IN RELATION TO FLOW

It was emphasized in the preceding discussion that the formation of blood in each body area of the embryo precedes the local demarcation of definitive blood vessels. As these focal collections of blood coalesce to form the primitive lacunar system and the blood within this system is increasingly set into motion by the rhythmic contractions of the heart, supplemented later by the intermittent contractions of skeletal muscles,[32] two significant phenomena become manifest. First, in those areas where flow becomes most active, the largest vessels develop from the mesenchyme surrounding the primitive lacunar system. Second, preferential pathways of flow become established, so that flow becomes constant in some channels but remains intermittent in others. The former phenomenon, observable during the development of the definitive arteries and veins during early embryogenesis.[10-13] and in adult life, requires no additional comment. The latter, more subtle phenomenon is observable in the various types of connections which become established between the arterial and venous systems during later life.

1. Thoroughfares, Capillaries, and Sinusoids

At the microscopic level, the study of living tissues by transillumination [26,37,40-47] has shown that three basic types of connections become established between the arteries and the veins: thoroughfare arteriovenous channels,[40-47] true arteriovenous capillaries,[40-44] and sinusoids.[26,37,40-47] In the thoroughfares, an arteriovenous pressure gradient is established such that arteriovenous flow is constantly maintained, irrespective of the flow status in the adjoining true arteriovenous capillaries or sinusoids.[26,37,40-47] In the true arteriovenous capillaries and sinusoids, which appear as side branching circuits to the thoroughfare arteriovenous channels, flow is only intermittently maintained and one group of capillaries or sinusoids is opening at a given time, then closing, to be supplanted by an adjacent group.[26,37,40-47] During the closed phase, the blood may lie static or reverse direction within a given capillary [40-44] or sinusoid.[26,37,46-47]

In conjunction with an increasing flow rate, an increasing order of histologic development is observable in these different types of channels.

a. Sinusoids

Owing to their irregular shapes,[19,25-27,31,36-37,46,48] relatively wide luminal diameters, [1,9,27,31,36-37,46,48] and intermittent flow,[26,37,45-47] the sinusoids probably rate lowest with respect to flow velocity. As pointed out by Bloom,[1] they seem to represent a primitive type of capillary. Similar to the mesenchyme-lined blood puddles of the primitive lacunar system, the sinusoids are not lined entirely by individual cells with definable cell membranes.[1] Instead, they remain partially lined by syncytial reticuloendothelium.[27,31,35-36,48] The individual nucleocytoplasmic territories* of this syncytium are heterogeneous, with some areas appearing endothelioid,[27,31,36,46] some containing intracytoplasmic reticular fibrils,[27,31,36,48] some containing engulfed particular matter,[27,31,35-36,48] and some ubiquitous, undifferentiated areas lacking all of these distinguishing features.[28,36,48] This syncytium is continuous with and inseparable from the reticulum forming the integral stroma of the hematopoietic organs.[31,36,48] No muscularis, basement membrane, nor any other definable barrier separates the syncytium from the reticulum surrounding the sinusoids.[31,36,48] Fine reticular fibrils identical and continuous with those of the reticulum traverse the cytoplasm, lending a fenestrated type of support to the sinusoidal walls.[48,50]

b. True Capillaries

Owing to their small, relatively uniform diameters,[1,9,40-44] the capillaries, at least during the flow phase of their intermittent

---

* Inasmuch as a syncytium is a multinucleated protoplasmic mass, seemingly an aggregation of several cells but without any perceptible cell outlines, the term "nucleocytoplasmic territory" [49] probably best describes individual areas consisting of nucleus and contiguous cytoplasm within such a multinucleated protoplasmic structure.

circulation, may be expected to have greater flow velocities than the sinusoids. The capillaries are lined predominantly,[1,9] but not necessarily entirely,[51,52] by common vascular endothelial cells. While these cells may appear fatter, less elongated, and more irregular than the common vascular endothelial cells in the vessels,[1,9,40-44] they differ from the reticuloendothelium of the the sinusoids in that they usually stand out as separate, individual cells with definite stainable boundaries after silver nitrate injection.[1] These individual common vascular endothelial cells are supported by basement membrane[50,53] and separated from the parenchymal cells of sundry tissues by loose (reticular) connective tissue.[1]

c. Thoroughfares and Vessels

The thoroughfare arteriovenous channels, as well as the arteries, veins, and main lymphatic ducts, demonstrate the most constant and rapid flow. All these channels are lined by common vascular endothelial cells which usually appear more uniform and elongated than the lining cells of the capillaries.[1,9] The endothelial cells, in turn, are supported by basement membrane and loose connective tissue[53] but, in addition, are separated from the parenchymal cells of the tissues by single or multiple layers of smooth muscle.[1,40-44] In contrast to the capillaries and sinusoids, innervation is demonstrable in the vessel walls.[54] The muscular layers and innervation are most highly developed in vessels proximal with respect to the heart and gradually thin out distally to become rudimentary at the points where the arteries and veins connect via the thoroughfare arteriovenous channels.[40-44]

2. The Physiologic Properties of the Various Vascular Channels

Just as the vessels, capillaries, and sinusoids differ in relation to flow and microscopic structure, they differ also with respect to certain physiologic properties.

a. Capacity for Differentiation

According to Maximow,[15,55] the common endothelium of vessels is a highly differentiated, specialized tissue lacking the capacity to differentiate further. The capillary endothelium is believed by some [11,15,32,56] to be identical with the vascular endothelium. On the other hand, it has been held by some [51,52] that certain cells lining the peripheral capillaries retain the full developmental potential of mesenchyme. A limited potential for development into histiocytoid cells is suggested by direct observation through transillumination.[56] Of those holding the first opinion, some [15,57] point out that the "adventitial cells," pericytes, or "active mesenchyma," adjacent to the capillary endothelium, retain full mesenchymal potential. It is pertinent to note that in some newly forming capillaries [17] and in some vascular beds outside of the blood-forming organs, the lining cells exist in the form of a syncytium,[9,17] rather than as simple isolated cells. It is debatable whether the components of a syncytium lining a circulatory channel should be called endothelium or be designated by a term connoting a lesser degree of differentiation. This is particularly true when one considers that some components of the syncytium may differentiate into monocytes and histiocytes.[58]

In contrast to the endothelium lining vessels and capillaries, there is ample evidence to suggest that the reticuloendothelium of the sinusoids retains within its syncytial heterogenous structure certain nucleocytoplasmic territories endowed with full mesenchymal potential for the development of blood cells, histiocytes, and common vascular endothelium.[31,35,36,48,55,59,61]

b. Reaction to Particulate Matter, Intravital Dyes, and Phagocytosis

The endothelium and walls of the organized vessels are relatively unaffected by the intravascular injection of particulate matter or intravital dyes.[35,36] In the capillaries, particulate matter, such as India ink, is often deposited in the intercellular substance between the capillary endothelial cells.[36,62] Intravital dyes and other proteins, to some extent, pass into the loose connective tissue and histiocytes outside the capillary endothelium but are incorporated to only a limited extent into the endothelial cells themselves.[35,36,56]

On the other hand, the syncytium lining the sinusoids shows great avidity for foreign particulate matter, intravital dyes, acid colloids, and effete cells. Such substances pass rapidly into the cytoplasm after intravenous injection in the case of the spleen, liver, and bone marrow, or after subcutaneous injection in the case of the lymph nodes.[35,36] In addition, these substances are noted to pass into the reticulum which underlies the immediate lining of the sinusoids.[36,46,48] After passage into the cytoplasm, many of these substances are digested and lose their identity as visible foreign material. They become incorporated into, and inseparable from, the relatively amorphous cytoplasm of the reticular syncytium.[36] Describing these reactions on the part of the tissue lining and surrounding the sinusoids, Aschoff[35] and Kiyono[63] popularized the concept of the reticuloendothelial system as a special apparatus primarily concerned with phagocytosis.

c. Permeability

The endothelium and supporting structures of vessels are relatively impermeable. The exchange of most solvents and solutes takes place at the capillary level.[56,64] The capillaries demonstrate an almost unlimited permeability to water and simple solutes such as oxygen, carbon dioxide, simple sugars, urea, and amino acids.[64] They are relatively impermeable to macromolecules the size of plasma proteins and, under normal conditions, are almost completely impermeable to suspended objects the size of platelets, erythrocytes, and leucocytes.[32,56,64] It is not certain whether escaping macromolecules pass through the intercellular cement substance, whether they pass through pores demonstrable in some capillary beds, or whether they are actively absorbed by pinocytosis.[1,9,50,56,65,66]

The sinusoidal reticuloendothelium, on the other hand, has been shown to be highly permeable to proteins such as intravital dyes, and to particulate matter which, as mentioned above under D, 2, b not only pass into the reticuloendothelium but also into the adjoining reticulum.[35,36,48] Furthermore, the intermittent permeability to nonmotile objects the size of erythrocytes is demonstrable in tissue sections[48] and in direct transillumination microscopy of living tissues.[46] In the latter type of study, according to MacKenzie,[46] Parpart,[47] and Whipple,[67] the intermittency and back-and-forth nature of such high permeability is clearly demonstrated. As will be emphasized in Chapter 25, this high order of permeability of the reticuloendothelium would appear to be of vital importance to the mechanics of hematopoiesis.

3. Summary and Conclusions

In this part of the analysis, the data from the literature are organized to suggest that as flow is induced in the mesenchymal anlage of the cardiovascular system by rhythmic cardiac and/or skeletal muscular contractions, the degree of mesenchymal differentiation into endothelium is proportional to the flow rate locally established. Where flow becomes constant and active, as in the definitive arteries, veins, and thoroughfare arteriovenous channels, the mesenchyme differentiates into common vascular endothelium. Where the flow remains intermittent and relatively sluggish, as in the sinusoids of liver and hemopoietic organs, the mesenchyme differentiates into reticuloendothelium, a tissue in part syncytially continuous with the reticulum, and a tissue more heterogeneous, less differentiated, more permeable, and more actively phagocytic than the common vascular endothelium.

Chapter 25

DISCUSSION

A. SPECIALIZATION WITHIN BLOOD AND BLOOD VESSELS

A S LIVING ORGANISMS increase in size, the distance between constituent cells becomes too great to allow for adequate nutrition by the simple diffusion of nutrient substances from the focal locations where the water, food, and oxygen are taken in. Consequently, in the higher forms of animal life, the hematopoietic organs and the cardiovascular system become increasingly developed to form and distribute the blood and lymph which, in turn, carry nutrient molecules to scattered locations from whence the molecules may finally diffuse onward into the tissues. As carriers of molecules, the blood and lymph are magnificently specialized so that oxygen, minerals, carbohydrates, amino acids, and fats are transported in concentrations much greater than can be supported in simple solution. The erythrocytes, for instance, increase the oxygen-carrying capacity of the blood sixty times per unit volume. The proteins of the blood and lymph not only carry amino acids, carbohydrates, and fats in concentrated form but also maintain the liquid state of the blood by osmotically counteracting the outward force exerted by intravascular hydrostatic pressure. In the latter capacity, the proteins also serve as carriers of water. Just as these blood and lymph constituents demonstrate such specialization with increasing phylogenetic development, so do the components of the hematopoietic and vascular systems show functional specialization.

The definitive vessels, owing to their constant flow, innervation, muscular walls, smooth common vascular endothelial cells, and low order of permeability, appear to be designed for the rapid transmission and controlled distribution of the blood and lymph. The thoroughfare arteriovenous channels with similar flow and structure appear to be designed not only for the controlled distribution of blood to the individual capillaries but also for the maintenance of a constant pressure gradient and flow between the arterial and venous systems. These two types of channels together appear to serve as a giant shunt apparatus which is capable not only of rapidly giving and receiving from portions of a capillary bed here and there during a given circuit, but also of sending to the lungs with each circuit the entire venous return at a rate roughly equal to the entire blood volume per minute (under resting conditions). The definitive vessels and thoroughfare arteriovenous channels, therefore, appear to be specialized not only for the rapid, controlled distribution of all that the blood contains but also for the rapid, constant maintenance of circulation necessary for the adequate oxygenation of a relatively large mass of tissue.

The true capillaries, owing to their widespread distribution, intermittent flow, lack of smooth muscle and innervation, their lining consisting predominantly of common vascular endothelial cells, and their intermediate order of permeability, appear to be specialized for the exchange of diffusible blood constituents between the intravascular compartment and the parenchyme of the tissue which the capillaries support. Since many more true capillaries are present than are open at any given time within a given capillary bed under resting conditions,[40-47] a tremendous capacity for variation of functional activity in accordance with variations in the functional activity of the adjacent parenchymal tissue is inherent in the architecture of the capillary bed.

The sinusoids, owing to their characteristic localization in the liver and hematopoietic organs,* their intermittent flow, their lack of muscular walls and innervation, their lack of basement membrane, their relatively undifferentiated character, their capacity for phagocytosis, and their high order of permeability, would appear to remain admirably adapted to the relatively primitive function of replenishing the intravascular blood and lymph from the extravascular hematopoietic tissue.

---

* It should be added that in the pituitary, adrenal, and pancreatic insular tissue, the endothelium functionally resembles the sinusoidal endothelium.[35,36] This functional similarity may be important to the intravascular secretion of macromolecular hormones from these glands.

B. WEAK FEATURES IN THE CURRENT CONCEPT OF VASCULOGENESIS AND HEMATOPOIESIS

According to the currently accepted concept of vasculogenesis and hematopoiesis,[68,69] the embryonal mesenchyme successively gives rise to isolated masses and cords of cells termed blood islands. Originally solid, the central portions of the blood islands give rise to plasma and primitive free-floating blood cells.* The peripheral cells of the blood islands become flattened endothelium. By the repetetive coalescence of the blood-filled spaces and the proliferative growth of endothelium, the blood vascular system is demarcated. Thus a system of closed vessels lined by endothelium is established. Once this system is established, all new vessels arise as endothelial outgrowths, with the lymphatics arising by sprouting from veins. The blood cells, then, continue to arise in the perivascular connective tissue which serves as the source of stem cells. The latter detach, proliferate, and ultimately migrate into the vascular system. This concept, while it explains the origin of the blood vessels and the blood cells, does not provide for the following:

1. How and from where the plasma arises after the vascular system is established.

2. How nonmotile blood cells, the cytoplasmic products of blood cells, and the plasma gain access to the closed vascular system.

3. How the lymphatics, upon arising from the venous endothelium, are filled with lymph instead of venous blood.

4. How aged cells and plasma proteins get out of or are removed from the closed vascular system to be reutilized in the manufacture of new blood.

The failure of accepted concepts to provide an adequate explanation for these specific problems is attributable to relative lack of agreement and/or knowledge in three basic parameters. First, the precise nature of the endothelium is not settled. Although it is recognized that the reticuloendothelium of the sinusoids differs from the common vascular endothelium lining

---

* The observation that the first plasma arises by dissolution of the mesenchymal syncytium is stated clearly only in Sabin's original descriptions.[11-13]

vessels, there are diverging opinions about whether or not the vascular system is really a closed system and whether the reticulo-endothelium should be considered as true endothelium. The crux of the argument here resides in the relationship which exists between the reticular connective tissue (reticulum), the reticulo-endothelium, and the common vascular endothelium, particularly with respect to which, if any, cells exist in a syncytial arrangement. Maximow and his followers [1,14,15,34,55] emphasized the universal distribution of reticular connective tissue throughout the body, as well as in hematopoietic organs; its analogous structure in all areas; and the persistence into adult life of undifferentiated mesenchyme within this tissue. While they admitted that individual cell outlines are often imperceptible, they were not convinced that the mesenchyme is a true syncytium. On the other hand, Downey,[29,31,35] Klemperer,[48,60] Jaffé,[36] and many of their European predecessors were convinced that the mesenchyme is a syncytium and that its counterpart in adult life, the reticulum, is also a syncytium. In addition, Downey [29,31] maintained and showed that the venous and lymphatic sinusoids are lined by flattened reticulum, not by ordinary endothelium. Aschoff,[35] when he described the phagocytic properties of the tissue lining sinusoids, deferred to Downey's opinion. Sabin [11,13] and her followers considered the mesenchyme to be a syncytium but related the tissue lining sinusoids more closely with endothelium than with the reticulum.

It is significant to note that the morphologic contributions of these and many other individuals were published before there was any clear discription of how blood actually flows through the sinusoids. Within a year of Maximow's death, Krogh [40] published the results of his observations on the microcirculation. Utilizing his methods of study, Clark and Clark,[17] Zweifach,[41,44] Knisely,[45] MacKenzie,[46] Bloch,[26] and Brånemark [37] confirmed Krogh's observations and expanded upon them. While these investigators agreed that the sinusoids and the true capillaries contain intermittent flow, whereas the vessels and thoroughfares contain constant flow, perhaps as a result of the preexisting controversy, they did not achieve agreement concerning the nature of the tissue lining the sinusoids. Realizing that this venerable argument is not soluble in an analysis such as this, it is hoped that a useful purpose is served by assuming a definite, although not currently popular, stand in the morphologic argument and attempting to show that the observed differences in the lining of sinusoids, capillaries, and vessels may be a function of the type of flow observed within them.

Second, the relationship of developing blood cells to the reticulum remains to be settled. While it is agreed that stem cells continue to differentiate from the reticulum forming the stroma of the hematopoietic organs, there is no clear indication at what stage of development these stem cells and their differentiated progeny normally detach from the stroma to become migratory cells. While some assume all the differentiated cells in hematopoietic organs to be cells floating more or less freely in tissue fluid outside of the blood vessels, others familiar with histology and pathology consider the cells to be relatively stationary within the reticular stroma or reticulum. As demonstrated by Isaacs,[70] the cells are quite incapable of migration until such time as this gelatinous connective tissue matrix undergoes a physicochemical change of state into a liquid which permits their free movement (a movement best described by the term "flow"). Again, while some may not be satisfied by answers provided in this analysis, not only is the mesenchymal and reticular connective tissue origin of the blood cells documented but also it is emphasized that blood cells continue their development in the reticulum surrounding sinusoids and in a very specific relation with the afferent and efferent vessels of various hemopoietic organs.

Third, it remains to be appreciated that all live cells are essentially gels whose dissolution will give rise to sols consisting of water and proteins. Application of this simple gel-sol principle to what will happen when cells shed cytoplasm or dissolve in the body results in identification of many of the cellular sources of the blood and lymph plasma, as outlined in Section 1, and as will be amplified further.

C. AN ANALYSIS OF BLOOD AND LYMPH SECRETION IN THE ADULT

A salient but poorly recognized feature of embryonal hemopoiesis and vasculogenesis is that the mesenchyme differentiates diffusely and dissolves to produce whole blood (or lymph) prior to the local establishment of definitive blood (or lymph) vessels. This sequence of events not only paves the way for the future development of the vascular system but also assures its initial filling with plasma, as well as with cells. Without this plasma, neither the cells nor the vessels would serve a useful purpose since the blood cells would lack a liquid medium in which to be suspended and flow, while the vessels would lack a liquid to contain and conduct.

Once the plasma and cells commence to flow under the impetus of striated muscle contractions and in definitive directions dictated by the orientation of valves,* common vascular endothelium flattens and differentiates out of the mesenchyme to expedite the conduction of intravascular fluid. With these developments definitive arteries, veins, and lymphatics take their origin, while the bulk of hemopoiesis shifts reciprocally from the yolk sac and general body mesenchyme into definitive hemopoietic organs, such as the liver, bone marrow, spleen, and other lymphoid organs. These hemopoietic organs, in turn, depending on their orientation toward specific extravascular sources of substrate and their relation toward afferent vessels (see Sect. 1; Chap. 18, A; and Chap. 25, C), become specialized to the production of specific varieties of circulating elements. The fact that hemopoiesis proceeds in the reticulum surrounding sinusoids, venous or lymphatic, lined by reticuloendothelium remains common to all definitive hemopoietic organs. In these sinusoids, flow remains inconstant in volume and direction while it evolutes to become relatively constant in definitive arteries, veins, and lymphatics surrounded by connective tissue and smooth muscle tunics of increasing thickness.

---

* Striated muscles, such as the heart, diaphragmatic, and skeletal muscles, impel the blood and lymph to flow. Heart valves direct the flow of arterial blood toward the periphery, while myriads of smaller valves direct the flow of venous blood and lymph toward the heart.

Thus, with the emphasis on fluids and their capacity to flow, some of the progressive events which take place during the simultaneous development of the interdependent vascular and hemopoietic systems can be outlined. Continuing the progression into adult life, flow remains of the essence, not only in the vascular system at large but also from the hematopoietic tissues into the vessels and from vessels into hemopoietic tissues. To maintain flow of the vital fluids for extended periods of time, three basic requirements must be met. First, production of whole blood and lymph in the reticulum must continue. Second, there must be a system for delivery of blood and lymph into the vascular system. Finally, there must be a system for reutilizing endogenous as well as exogenous substrate for hemopoiesis.

1. Continued Production of Whole Blood and Lymph in Hemopoietic Organs

In the reticulum of hemopoietic organs, blood cells are produced via two pathways [2,29,71]: (a) by direct differentiation from reticular cells and (b) by division of partially differentiated cells of definitive types.

Similarly, there are two pathways whereby plasma may be produced: (a) by direct dissolution of the reticulum and (b) by dissolution of cytoplasmic droplets shed from partially differentiated cells of definitive types.

The first, or direct, pathway of plasma production was described by Isaacs,[70] who showed that the reticular matrix of the hemopoietic organs is a gel and that this gel dissolves when mature blood cells are released. Although he did not ascribe particular significance to the products of matrical dissolution, phsyico-chemical principles dictate that the dissolution of a gel will yield a sol. Because the gelatinous reticular matrix, like the ground substance elsewhere,[53] is made up of water and polymerized, relatively low molecular weight proteins, one may expect its dissolution to yield a sol consisting of water and relatively low molecular weight, osmotically important proteins.

The second, less direct pathway of plasma production (already described in Sect. 1 and elsewhere[6]) is through release of cytoplasmic droplets (formerly called hyaline bodies [6,29,72]) from various kinds of developing mononuclear cells. These droplets, in turn, disperse and dissolve to release plasma consisting of water and a variety of high-molecular-weight,[6,73,74] electrophoretically slow-moving,[73,74] immunologically reactive,[73,74] nutritionally important [6,75] free extracellular proteins. The process appears entirely similar to the secretion of milk by the release of cytoplasmic droplets from mammary (acinar) epithelial cells (see Figs. 13 and 14).

While it is not clear at almost any stage of development or later life precisely what quantities of cells and plasma are derived directly from the reticulum, as opposed to quantities derived from partially differentiated cells of various types, it seems clear that in order to flow from the reticulum into the vascular system and onward, the cells and plasma must be secreted together, i.e. in the form of whole blood or lymph.

2. A System for Delivery of Blood and Lymph into the Vascular System

The transfer of newly formed blood or lymph into the intravascular compartment involves, in addition to the movement of motile blood cells, the movement of nonmotile formed elements, the movement of water, and the movement of many substances of varying size, varying molecular weight and therefore varying capacities for independent motility by means of diffusion, Brownian movement, and capillary attraction. As indicated by Isaacs,[70] dissolution of the gelatinous matrix in which the cells take their origin supplies a liquid medium capable of carrying both motile and nonmotile formed elements into the sinusoids. It should be added to his observation that dissolution of the matrix and dissolution of cytoplasmic droplets shed from developing cells will result in the formation of sols whose proteins, by virtue of their colloid osmotic properties, will enable new blood or lymph to hold water and therefore maintain fluidity against the force exerted by intravascular hydrostatic pressure.

Since new blood or lymph are thus established as fluids osmotically capable of retaining water, they may actually move by flowing into venous or lymphatic sinusoids when conditions of intrasinusoidal hydrostatic pressure and reticuloendothelial permeability are favorable. Such favorable conditions are bound to occur during that phase of the intermittent sinusoidal flow cycle when intrasinusoidal hydrostatic pressure falls, flow ceases, the intrasinusoidal blood or lymph stagnates, the local ogygen tension falls, pH falls, carbon dioxide tension rises, and the permeability of the sinusoidal reticuloendothelium accordingly approaches its maximum.[45,56,76]

3. A System for Reutilizing Endogenous, as Well as Exogenous, Circulating Material for Hemopoiesis

It is of primary importance to continual blood formation that the high order of permeability in sinusoidal reticuloendothelium is bidirectional. The same physiological conditions which permit newly formed cells and plasma to flow from the reticulum into the sinusoids with reversed pressure gradients and flow allow circulating cells and plasma to flow from the sinusoids into the reticulum. As already mentioned, the capacity of elements lining sinusoids to incorporate acid colloids and foreign particulate matter was demonstrated long ago, with the early histologists pointing out simultaneously that these substances, moreover, disperse quite rapidly into the extrasinusoidal reticulum.[35,36,48] Again, evidence for passage of endogenous, nonmotile particles as large as erythrocytes from the circulation into the extravascular reticulum of various lymphoid organs seems well documented in histologic studies,[31,36,48] while the bidirectional flow of blood cells and plasma to and from the reticulum of the living spleen has been observed by transillumination.[46]

One may then envision acid colloids, particulate matter, blood cells, plasma, and their large molecular constituents as nondiffusible forms of molecular substrate which flow intermittently from the circulation into the reticulum to be reutilized selectively for hemopoiesis. That reutilization, indeed, takes place there can be documented in several ways, singly or in combination, as follows.

1. Histiocytes appear to digest dye-labeled acid colloids, mi-

mation from disintegrating (immunologically competent, memory-retaining) small lymphocytes to other mononuclear cells involved during earlier stages of the sequential cellular response.

4. Summary and Conclusions

Here the data are organized to indicate that the mesenchyme of the early embryo and its adult counterpart, the reticulum, produce circulating cells and plasma by identical mechanisms. The cells are produced by direct differentiation, while the plasma is produced directly by dissolution. Myriads of additional cells arise by division of partially differentiated cells, while a quantities of additional plasma arises by dissolution of cytoplasmic droplets shed from differentiating mononuclear cells. As in early embryonal hemopoiesis, dissolution of the gelatinous reticular matrix and dissolution of cytoplasmic droplets provide sols which enable newly formed blood or lymph to flow and to osmotically retain the water which enables flow. The principal difference between the embryonal and the adult form of hemopoiesis appears to lie in the fact that the former is mainly oriented toward vasculogenesis, whereas the latter is oriented toward the replenishment of an established vascular system. While the early embryonal mesenchyme utilizes relatively invisible and diffusible molecular substrate from the yolk sac entoderm to establish a vascular system filled with blood, the reticulum must continue in a position where it can utilize the nondiffusible, as well as the diffusible, contents of the system in order to replenish it. It is suggested that the high order of intermittent permeability of the reticuloendothelium lining sinusoids not only permits the intravascular movement of newly formed blood or lymph but also permits the escape of the nondiffusible contents of the system, such as effete cells and endogenous and foreign proteins so that these substances can be digested within histiocytes and reutilized in the production of new blood or lymph.

D. AN ANALYSIS OF HEMATOPOIETIC TISSUE SPECIALIZATION AS A FUNCTION OF AFFERENT SUBSTRATE MOVEMENT

While the term "hemopoiesis" is sometimes used to describe the bone marrow's activity in producing erythrocytes, the blood is really a composite of the plasma and cells secreted from several hemopoietic tissues, including the bone marrow, the spleen, scattered lymphatic tissues, and the mesenchymal component of the liver. It is the product of central mixing of formed elements and plasma secreted into the venous effluent of the marrow; into the portal venous effluent from the spleen, gut, and liver; and into the lymph effluent from nodes and diffusely arranged lymphatic tissues in many portions of the body. Inasmuch as all hematopoietic tissues commence their development similarly,[14] all are capable of producing diverse hemic elements similarly during embryonal and adult life,[14,24,60,61,87] all have a similar reticular stroma in which the hemic elements arise,[1,14,15,34,36,48,55,60] and all contain sinusoids lined by reticuloendothelium,[1,14,31,35,36,48,60] the foregoing analysis of intravascular secretion is intended to be applicable to all. As the embryo grows into the adult, however, the ultimate normal pattern of development is such that each tissue becomes specialized to the production of a relatively limited variety of hemic elements. This specialization appears to occur in association with the local development of specific types of afferent and efferent vessels and the reliance on specific pathways whereby additional molecular substrate necessary for hemopoiesis are acquired (see Figs. 1-3). On the basis of afferent vascular supply and additional afferent pathways, the hematopoietic tissues may be subdivided into five separate, interdependent categories.

1. Tissues Supplied Only by Afferent Arteries

The bone marrow and spleen are the outstanding examples in the category of tissues supplied only by afferent arteries. These tissues receive the molecular substrate necessary for growth and function entirely via arterioles and arteriovenous sinusoids. The extravascular hematopoietic tissue in each organ receives readily diffusible substances such as water, oxygen, glucose, and amino acids via the arterioles. In addition to these diffusible substances, the hematopoietic tissue receives and visably assimilates [36] relatively nondiffusible substances such as formed elements and proteins via the arteriovenous sinusoids. The principal difference between the bone marrow and the spleen appears to reside not in the type of afferent blood supply but in the quantity. Whereas the bone marrow has a small arterial supply [28] and is maintained in a low oxygen concentration,[88] the splenic tissue has a large arterial supply [28,48] and is maintained in a high oxygen concentration.[89]

The marrow tissue, residing within a restricted space within cancellous bone (where a low arterial flow and low oxygen tension can be maintained quite remote from the external environment), supplies local conditions best suited to the production of erythrocytes, granulocytes, platelets,[28] and a plasma whose volume and protein constituents (aside from myeloma proteins) remain to be measured with precision. (The role of the periarteriolar lymphoid tissue in producing some of this plasma and the flushing function of latter is outlined in Chap. 18, A, 5).

On the other hand, the splenic hemopoietic tissue, being maintained in a relatively high concentration of oxygen, provides local conditions best suited to the production of lymphocytes [28,90] and a plasma whose volume and protein constituents (other than immune globulins) remain to be measured. In addition, because the spleen is endowed with a relatively large arterial supply and because it is situated in the peritoneal cavity where rapid volume changes are permissible,[46,91] it is admirably suited to the storage of blood,[91-92] the histiocytic destruction of relatively large quantities of circulating formed elements [92,93] and proteins,[36,47,77] and the storage of proteins within its relatively large mononuclear cell population.[75] While the spleen's roles in the storage and destruction of blood elements are well recognized, it remains to be appreciated that whatever is destroyed must be reutilized, that splenic mononuclear cells synthesize proteins at a relatively rapid rate,[94] and that they are eminently capable of releasing them by cytoplasmic shedding or by dissolving at a rapid rate.[75] Credit should be accorded White and Dougherty [75] for showing that the spleen constitutes one of the largest and most labile of protein reservoirs in the body and that its lymphocytes shed their cytoplasm or dissolve to release their proteins for nutritive purposes in other tissues, particularly during starvation. As already mentioned in Chapters 11 and 18, A, filling of the splenic protein reservoir is fostered by increased splanchnic blood flow each time a meal containing protein is absorbed.[46] Increased splanchnic flow assures splenic receipt of an important share of the chyle circulated from intestinal lymphoid tissue.

Reduced to simplest terms, then, the prime function of the bone marrow is to utilize diffusible and relatively nondiffusible molecular substrate from its relatively sparse arterial circulation to produce plasma and formed elements (mostly erythrocytes) which are diluted into the systemic venous circulation and which flow centrally to pick up oxygen in the pulmonary capillary bed. A prime function of the spleen, on the other hand, is to reutilize diffusible and nondiffusible molecular substrate from its rich arterial circulation to produce plasma and formed elements (principally lymphocytes) which are diluted into the portal venous circulation * and which flow centrally, carrying diverse forms of nourishment first to the hepatic capillary bed and subsequently to remaining capillary beds. Such prime functions are trophic with the marrow being specialized largely to produce elements containing hemoglobin, a protein which facilitates the transport of oxygen to capillary beds beyond the pulmonary circuit. The spleen would appear specialized largely to the production of mononuclear cells which ingest, digest, reutilize, store, and release diverse proteins so that the latter can be used again for growth first in the liver and subsequently in other organs. Incidentally, as the spleen breaks down large quantities of hemoglobin (as well as proteins emanating from diverse blood cells), its situation as the "regional node" to the marrow and as an imminent protein supply for the liver are of profound medical significance.

---

* Dilution of plasma and cells of splenic origin into a relatively voluminous portal venous effluent undoubtedly makes it difficult to measure splenic output directly and to compare splenic output with that of other hemopoietic organs.

2. Tissues Supplied by Afferent Arteries and Lymphatics

The widely dispersed, encapsulated lymph nodes are the examples in this category. Via rich networks of small arterioles [34] their follicular (cortical) portions receive diffusible and relatively non-diffusible molecular substrate from the circulating blood via rich networks of small arterioles (as outlined on pp. 171-178). Via their maze-like lymphatic sinusoidal systems (whose development is described on pp. 320-322), the medullary portions of the nodes not only receive diffusible substrate, but also receive and ostensibly assimilate [32,35,36] relatively nondiffusible substances effluent from the peripheral tissues to which they are regional. As emphasized by Drinker and Yoffey,[32] the peripheral lymph which emanates from the peripheral connective tissues supporting the arteriovenous capillaries and the parenchymal cells of all definitive organs is always interrupted by a passage through nodes on its course toward the central lymphatics.

Therefore, if the nodes reutilize some of the diffusible and relatively nondiffusible molecules from their afferent arteries and from their afferent (peripheral) lymphatics, one may state simply that a prime function of the nodes is to produce central lymph which is diluted into that portion of peripheral lymph which remains after passage through the nodes. The production of central lymph involving the production of plasma as well as cells, the wide immunologic and trophic consequences of nodal lymph production are outlined in Chapter 18. It should suffice to mention here that all lymph nodes other than those in the gastrointestinal mesenteries are oriented toward nonabsorptive or external surfaces and therefore primarily concerned with the reutilization of substances emanating from cells concerned with vital processes other than the absorption of food.

The foregoing simple, vitalistic concept of lymph formation in the nodes, of course, is foreign to current concepts which maintain that lymph is formed primarily by filtration (see Chap. 28). Having shown that quantities of circulating plasma proteins filter from the arteriovenous capillaries into peripheral and central lymphatics, Drinker, Yoffey, and others considered the nodes to be filters which trap foreign proteins, instead of quantitatively important sources of central lymph. Under the assumption that all the plasma albumin and most of its globulins are formed in the liver (presumably by hepatic parenchymal cells; see p. 355), the lymphatic apparatus (including the nodes) is still envisioned as a system whose primary function is to absorb proteins from peripheral tissues and to return to the blood circulation those plasma proteins which have filtered out in the periphery. This is an accurate concept, but it does not cover how these proteins are absorbed or what they are ultimately used for. Moreover, it is based on a shaky assumption coupled with a leaky theory.

The Shaky Assumption. While there is histologic evidence to indicate that the mononuclear cells in the nodes and in other lymphoid organs secrete water and free extracellular proteins into central lymphatics by shedding cytoplasm or dissolving [81,82,95] (and see Sect. 1), morphologic evidence is lacking that the parenchymal cells forming the bulk of the normal liver secrete any definitive product other than bile and some of the muco-proteins which it contains (see p. 357).

A Leaky Theory. The filtration theory explains how proteins of differing molecular weight and varying molecular configuration are differentially filtered through the endothelium (or through pores between endothelial cells). This theory does not explain how filtered proteins (which diffuse more slowly than water) not only filter through intervening tissues into lymphatics but do so at rates which must exceed that of water if the water is to be osmotically drawn into lymph capillaries at the expense of surrounding connective tissues. Moreover, the filtration theory fails to take into account the reutilization of leaking proteins in diverse tissues (see p. 363) and fails to take into account the intravascular secretion of a significant quantity of osmotically active protein by any tissue other than the liver.

Insofar as the nodes are concerned, they merely lie in a suitable position to either trap or pass on proteins which enter via peripheral lymph, while adding free extracellular proteins and cells shed from indigenous cell populations. The central lymph, then, will contain a mixture of proteins from two sources: the peripheral tissues and the nodal cell populations. Inasmuch as the latter ostensibly shed relatively basophilic, pyroninophilic, high-molecular-weight, globular proteins (see Figs. 4–27), one must assume that relatively large quantities of proteins of this variety are added, an assumption which is borne out by comparing peripheral and central lymph with respect to total protein content and albumin: globulin ratios (see Chap. 8).

Finally, it should be mentioned that the nodes constitute one of the easiest areas in which to study lymph formation under the microscope, owing to the fact that they contain many mononuclear cells, while dilution of erythrocytes into their sinsuoids is normally minimal (see Figs. 9–12).

3. Tissues Supplied by Arterioles and Parenchymal Cells Involved with Absorption

The outstanding examples in the category of tissues supplied by arterioles and parenchymal cells involved with absorption are the thymus gland and the lymphoid tissue of the intestine. Since each has been considered at some length in earlier portions of the text, only pointed comments on their phylogenetic or embryologic development as they relate to ultimate function will be recounted here.

The epithelial portion of the thymus gland takes its embryologic origin from gill entoderm, a parenchymal cell layer concerned with the absorption of oxygen in lower orders of vertebrates which swim, feed, and respire under water. During vertebrate evolution, as well as during mammalian embryogenesis, as the animal prepares to breathe air and walk on land, the gill entoderm invaginates into the lower neck to become the stranded epithelium of the thymus, thyroid, and parathyroid glands. As outlined in Section 2, the stranded thymic epithelium takes on an endocrine function which greatly enhances lymphocytopoiesis and the ability of the neonate to survive birth and to thrive while breathing air on land. Interestingly enough, other epithelial remnants from the gill entoderm, such as the thyroid and parathryoid epithelium, produce hormones which, respectively, modulate the amount of oxygen consumed, and modulate the growth of bones which form a rigid thorax and enable the animal to walk on land. Having nothing more to do with the absorption of oxygen, the stranded thymic epithelial cells produce a hormone which accelerates its utilization for DNA synthesis and growth in lymphocytes (possibly by catalysis of oxidative chain phosphorylizations). As a result, close to the stranded thymic epithelium and in a tissue environment preferentially treated with respect to oxygenation during the evolution of the gill arches into the principal outflow tracts of the heart, extraordinarily large numbers of small lymphocytes grow out of the thymic mesenchyme. Thus a lymphoepithelial organ which grows to become one of the largest organs in the body at the time of birth in mammals is formed from stranded gill epithelium and mesenchyme which differentiates primarily into lymphoid elements. Subsequently, this lymphoepithelial organ involutes or shrinks gradually in relation to total body mass, and in so doing releases a hormone and small lymphocytes (or the products of their disintegration) to enchance the growth and development of remaining lymphoid organs in the body. During stress when tissue oxygenation is prone to be particularly critical, an increased release of adrenal glucocorticoids incites the gland to shrink extremely rapidly through lymphocytolysis. Relatively large quantities of small lymphocyte desoxyribonucleic acids, compounds extremely rich in high-energy phosphate bonds linked with nucleosides are given up, then. Finally, during a persons childhood or later life, this gland is a definitive lymphoid organ which utilizes diffusible, and (owing to a relative lack of sinusoids) relatively small quantities of nondiffusible, molecular substrate to produce a hormone and small lymphocytes. The latter flow forth together, to enhance DNA synthesis and growth in remaining lymphoid organs, so that these organs, in turn, may perform their definitive immunologic and trophic functions more efficiently.

The intestinal lymphoid tissue is derived from the mesenchyme which underlies and supports the yolk sac entoderm. Here, the first whole blood of the developing embryo is derived (as utilization of the yolk for body growth commences). In invertebrates and in lower orders of vertebrates, it comprises either

the only or the principal lymphoid organ in the body and occupies a position increasingly close to the digestive tube, as one
descends the phylogenetic scale.[7] When the land-roving vertebrate
hatches from the egg or emerges from the womb and starts feeding, this segment of the mesenchyme undergoes hypertrophy to
become one of the largest but most diffusely arranged lymphoid
tissues in the body. During starvation, this segment of the lymphoid tissue mass shrinks rapidly. With each meal containing
protein or protein and fat, it undergoes hypertrophy at a rapid
rate, owing to cellular hyperplasia.[32,80,96] The reticulum or reticular connective tissue here supports not only aggregates of
growing mononuclear cells, but also the entodermal cells lining
the intestine. A rich, arching arterial network supplies oxygen
and other highly diffusible forms of molecular substrate and does
so in increased quantities during the absorption of a meal containing protein. No afferent lymphatics are demonstrable, and
histiocytes are relatively infrequent under normal conditions.
Instead, all diffusible and nondiffusible substrate coming from
sources other than the afferent arterioles come from the entodermal cells concerned with the absorption of food. Moreover,
all diffusible and nondiffusible molecules absorbed via the
intestinal mucosal cells must first pass through this layer before
gaining access to centrally oriented lymphatics (lacteals) or into
the radicles of the portal vein. In this position, the diffuse
intestinal lymphoid tissue is admirably located to utilize diffusible
and nondiffusible substrate from the entodermal cells concerned
with absorption as well as from the afferent arterioles to produce
a form of lymph known as chyle. This chyle flows centrally
(with interruptions in mesenteric lymph nodes) to constitute
the bulk of lymph in the thoracic duct, especially after a meal.
The chyle consists of water, salts, carbohydrates, amino acids,
proteins, and lymphocytes and is particularly prone to be milky,
owing to a relatively high concentration of newly absorbed high-
molecular-weight fats linked to proteins (lipoproteins). Conveyed via the thoracic duct, this chyle flows into the onward
through the blood vascular system, to be distributed to other
lymphoid and nonlymphoid organs in volumes which depend on

rates of arterial flow to each organ. Here the various constituents of chyle may be reutilized, singly, separately, selectively, or collectively, for growth.

4. Tissues Supplied by Afferent Arteries and Afferent Veins

The lungs and liver of adult mammals are unique in that their capillary beds are supplied mostly by venous blood of relatively low oxygen tension carried in via the pulmonary artery and portal vein, respectively. Their intrinsic arterial blood supply seems relatively small in comparison. Critically involved with absorption, the lungs take in oxygen, while the liver is linked indirectly to the intake of food (see p. 354). Around the small arteries supplying these organs with fully oxygenated blood, i.e. the bronchial and hepatic arterioles, normally one finds organized lymphoid tissue in the form of peribronchial nodes and diffusely arranged in the portal triads, respectively. While the lymphoid development of mesenchyme in the lungs is potentially of great interest, only the functional development of liver mesenchyme will be considered here, particularly as related to the influx of food.

As seen in the normal mammalian adult, ultimate mesenchymal development seems relatively complex owing to attenuation of the mesenchymal layer by growth of adjacent parenchymal cells.* With focus only on mesenchymal components, one may envision hepato-cellular consistency as in Figure 1b. Having developed mostly to consist of histiocytes and macrophages (Kupffer cells), the mesenchymal layer of the liver seems particularly specialized to ingest and digest endogenous cell remnants and free extracellular proteins of endogenous, as well as exogenous origin.[27] Nevertheless, the mesenchymal portion of the liver constitutes a reticular stroma of many parts, all dependent upon portal venous blood and hepatic arterial blood for the substrate essential to continued growth and function, not only locally but also in adjacent parenchymal cells.

Physically supporting the blood vessels, lymph vessels, and the hepatic parenchymal cells, yet separating them from one another,[1,27]

---

* Also, the degree of hepatic mesenchymal attenuation if related (inversely) to local hemopoietic activity (see pp. 354–355).

the hepatic mesenchymal layer grows in a position to mediate all macromolecular and micromolecular exchanges in between. While the ingestion, digestion, and incorporation of portions of cells and macromolecules brought in via the hepatic artery and portal vein are the most obvious metabolic functions of the hepatic mesenchymal cells, particularly those disposed in the sinusoidal regions, the manner of disposition of smaller molecules is less obvious, but no less important.

For instance, some of the macromolecules and many micromolecules from the afferent blood circulation are incorporated into the mesenchymal layer to support growth. Some macromolecules and micromolecules from the afferent blood circulation filter through the mesenchymal layer into the hepatic lymphatics and into the hepatic parenchymal cells. Moreover, some of the macromolecules and micromolecules, initially incorporated into the cells of the mesenchymal layer, are excreted (or secreted) onward into the hepatic venules, hepatic lymphatics, or into the adjacent parenchymal cells.

Along with molecules excreted from the mesenchymal layer, the hepatic parenchymal cells receive molecules filtered through from the afferent blood circulation. Many of these molecules, then, may be selectively reutilized to sustain protoplasmic growth in the parenchymal cells, be excreted into bile, or be returned via diffusion into the mesenchymal layer.

Those molecules returned to the mesenchymal layer from parenchymal cells, in turn, may be reutilized for local cellular growth, along with molecules coming in via the afferent blood circulation. Or they may diffuse onward into the lymphatic spaces of Dissé, or into the hepatic venous sinusoids to be circulated and reutilized elsewhere. Finally, of those molecules reutilized for local growth in the mesenchymal layer, some may be excreted (or secreted) by clasmatosis into the hepatic lymphatics or into the efferent veins of the liver.

In this manner some of the complex molecular circuitry in the liver may be analyzed, particularly as one concentrates on the cells comprising the mesenchymal layer. It should be obvious, however, that liver function does not depend solely on the activity of one particular kind of cell, or any definitive layer of cells. Instead, it depends on the integrated activity of all cellular components, particularly as all relate to the afferent and efferent circulation. Therefore, in assessing liver function one must continue analysis in terms of the cooperative activity between mesenchymal components and parenchymal cells which conjointly accomplish the following:

1. The breakdown of heme pigments linked to proteins (conjugated pigments), such that some of their portions may be resorbed for reutilization, while others may be excreted into the bile ducts.[97]

2. The breakdown of circulating cells and cell remnants, various free extracellular proteins, and many of their amino acid constituents into ammonia, followed by conversion of some into urea which may diffuse back into the circulation or into the bile ducts.[97]

3. The breakdown of cellular and free extracellular proteins into their amino acid moieties, followed by oxidation, reduction, deamination, or transamination of the latter (along with diffusing amino acids from the circulation) into compounds which can be reutilized both locally and in other parts of the body for cellular growth upon release by diffusion from the cells engaged in the respective processes.[97]

4. The breakdown of circulating cellular and free extracellular proteins (as well as amino acids and fats diffusing from the circulation) into simple compounds which are resynthesized into glucose which, in turn, may diffuse into the circulation or be stored locally as glycogen.[97]

If the liver fails to perform some or all of these functions (as may be observed clinically in infectious hepatitis, or in Laennec's cirrhosis), one commonly sees failure of normal growth in remaining tissues, as evidenced by weight loss, wasting, or atrophy; failure of adequate blood hemoglobin production by cells in the bone marrow [98]; and failure of adequate blood plasma protein production [97,99,100] irrespective of the cells or organs wherein these free extracellular proteins are produced.[101]

Thus the hepatic mesenchyme and parenchyme are quantitatively and critically involved in turning over the constituents of circulating cells, free extracellular proteins, amino acids, fats, and carbohydrates. They may be envisioned as tissues conjointly concerned in maintaining balance in the effluent hepatic venous, lymphatic, and subsequent confluent systemic concentration of all such entities through utilization of that which enters the liver via the relatively large portal vein and the small hepatic artery. Therefore, during starvation, in order to maintain stability in circulating systemic concentrations of circulating cells, free extracellular proteins, amino acids, fats, and carbohydrates, the liver may be expected to turn over relatively large quantities of cells, free extracellular proteins, amino acids, fats, and carbohydrates emanating from other tissues, especially the shrinking spleen which drains solely * and directly into the liver (see Chaps. 5 and 18, A). Similarly, if the diet is inadequate with respect to given proteins, amino acids, fats, carbohydrates or other known substances (such as vitamins), through the concerted action of its mesenchymal and parenchymal cells, the liver may be expected to compensate the circulating systemic deficit by turning over cells, free extracellular proteins, amino acids, fats, carbohydrates, and other substances from the same proximal and more distant sources.

It is embryologically and phylogenetically pertinent to reiterate here that in all vertebrates, the liver takes its origin conjointly from the mesenchyme of the septum transversum and the primitive gut entoderm while the former is being invaded by cells budding and becoming stranded from the latter.[8,10] This differentiation transpires as the yolk is used up and the developing vertebrate must prepare to take its subsequent nourishment by mouth (as in all oviparous species) or from the placenta (as in mammals). With the utilization of the yolk to create plasma and blood cells in the subentodermal growing mesenchyme, the establishment of rudimentary vessels through fusion of mesenchymal spaces containing plasma and free blood cells, and the propulsion of this whole blood via definitive vessels from the anlage

---

* Although the intestine drains via the portal system into the liver; also, it drains via centrally oriented lymphatics into the thoracic duct. Moreover, both the venous and lymphatic drainage from the intestine are reduced during starvation, as compared with the postprandial state.

of the gut to the budding, stranding entodermal cells (see Chap. 24), the liver takes on its relatively adult appearance as a parenchymal organ increasingly dominated by its own entodermal parenchymal cells, instead of its blood-forming mesenchymal cells. Thus demarcated as a separate, definitive organ, the liver continues to grow, characteristically maintaining connections to its entodermal anlage via the portal vein (derived from mesenchyme) and the bile ducts (derived from stranded entodermal cells). As an appendage to the gut (in ovulates) and to the placenta (in mammals), the liver remains a quantitatively important blood-forming organ in many of the lower vertebrates and, during the middle third of gestation, in most mammals.[7,8,10] However, its hemopoietic importance relative to extrahepatic sites of blood formation would seem to decrease with ascent of the phylogenetic scale, with increasing gestational development in mammals, and with an increasing arteriovenous oxygen difference in many species.[28] Thus we see during the embryogenesis of the liver, the development of a direct appendage to the gut and the development of an organ which, during alimentation, can augment the digestive function of the latter by secreting bile to aid in the emulsification and subsequent absorption of fat. During starvation, it may be envisioned as an organ admirably suited to compensate for the lack of absorption, doing so by releasing some of its own glycogen and proteins and by turning over proteins from other tissues to maintain constant concentrations of circulating simple compounds, such as glucose and amino acids, as outlined above.

Although neither the production of blood cells (see Chap. 28), nor the production of the blood plasma are considered to be prime functions of the adult mammalian liver, it is assumed currently that liver cells, particularly its parenchymal cells, are the principal source of the circulating plasma proteins. This assumption is based on the following clinical and experimental observations:

1. Individuals having parenchymal liver disease, such as Laennec's cirrhosis or viral hepatitis, often demonstrate hypoalbu-

minemia coupled with diminution in the total concentration of circulating plasma proteins.[99]

2. In individuals having cirrhosis of the liver or hepatitis, there is relative inability to form serum albumin, even when large quantities of proteins are fed. Inasmuch as these individuals may have positive nitrogen balance, thus attesting to their ability to synthesize and store proteins, the data suggest a direct relationship between alterations in liver function and the failure to maintain a normal level of circulating albumin.[99]

3. The hepatectomized animal (with portal vein, hepatic artery, and efferent hepatic lymphatics, therefore, ligated) appears relatively unable to synthesize circulating plasma proteins.[99,100]

4. In animals having the liver partially excluded from the portal circulation (via an Eck fistula which drains portal venous blood into the inferior vena cava), there is diminished capacity to replete plasma proteins after removing plasma proteins from the body (plasmapheresis).[99]

5. Prolonged limitation of protein intake not only diminishes the level of serum albumin but also is accompanied by histologic changes in hepatic cells, such as fatty metamorphesis and atrophic changes.[99]

6. The livers of rats appear to synthesize all the plasma albumin and 80 percent of the plasma globulin, as judged by perfusion of isolated livers with isotope labeled amino acids, whereas the remaining eviscerated carcasses appear to synthesize relatively little during the course of similar experiments.[3-5]

7. Liver slices in tissue culture can synthesize albumin and incorporate ^{14}C-labeled glycine into the proteins of the cultured cells.[102] Moreover, the observed cellular rate of incorporation of ^{14}C into protein is calculated compatible with the normal rate of plasma protein replacement.[100]

These observations, although they indicate that the liver plays a central role in adult mammalian protein metabolism, shed relatively little light on which cells in the liver, the mesenchymal cells or the parenchymal cells, actually secrete the plasma proteins. Attacking first the assumption that the parenchymal cells secrete the bulk of the plasma proteins, the following items are pertinent.

Both phylogenetically and embryologically, prior to the development of the liver, the mesenchyme directly underlying the yolk sac entoderm and the mesenchyme progressively more distant gives rise not only to the blood cells but also to the plasma in which they are suspended (see Chap. 24).

During and following the embryologic demarcation of the liver in the mesenchyme of the septum transversum, the mesenchyme here and that of most remaining body areas continues to give rise to whole blood or to lymph, consisting of plasma as well as cells (see Sect. 1 and Chap. 24).

Separated from the circulating blood and lymph by a definitive, albeit thin and relatively permeable layer of mesenchymal connective tissue, if the hepatic parenchymal cells were to secrete the bulk of the plasma proteins as isolated compounds, the osmotic effect would be to attract the bulk of the circulating plasma water to the parenchymal-mesenchymal interface. Thus, the colloid osmotic effect would be to deplete the adjacent mesenchymal connective tissue and the circulatory system of water, instead of repleting the latter with plasma.

Although the hepatic parenchymal cells, like all living cells, are capable of synthesizing protoplasmic proteins, histologic evidence remains to be presented that they secrete any large quantitiy of their protoplasm or any large quantity of free extracellular proteins (other than the mucoproteins in bile[104]). The histologic evidence still stands (as summarized in Sect. 1) that mesenchymal cells, particularly reticular cells, histiocytes, and macrophages, are capable of secreting protoplasm or free extracellular proteins in quantity. One need only remark that the mesenchymal component of the liver contains relatively large numbers of the latter and that the remaining definitive blood forming organs contain many, also (see Fig. 1 b).

With respect to the rate at which hepatic parenchymal cells synthesize protoplasmic proteins, it is well known that they normally synthesize nuclear proteins at a very slow rate, as evidenced by their low order of mitotic activity and their slow rate of utilization of labeled DNA precursors. As evidenced by their low order of cytoplasmic basophilia and pyroninophilia, as compared with the mass (see Sect. 1) of plasmacytes and large and medium-sized lyphocytes in the definitive hemopietic organs, one may assume that their rate of cytoplasmic protein synthesis is relatively slow, also. Therefore, whether or not the parenchymal cells actually shed protoplasmic proteins as droplets, in the form of whole cells or in the form of isolated proteins, into the circulatory system, the rate at which they synthesize such proteins is not indicative of a relatively important intravascular contribution in comparison with the mesenchymal mononuclear cells in the definitive hemopoietic organs.

With respect to the quantities of plasma or specific plasma proteins normally secreted by the liver as a whole or by any of its cells, the following items are pertinent.

In the adult mammalian liver, the bulk of the cells are parenchymal cells. In none of the aforementioned clinical, surgical, tissue culture, or perfusion experiments are the role of the hepatic parenchymal cells singled out or distinguished as being separate from that of the hepatic mesenchymal cells. Because the bulk of the cells are parenchymal cells, it is merely *assumed* that they secrete the bulk of the plasma proteins under the conditions of the experiment.

Almost every areolar connective tissue in the body, and especially the reticular stroma of the definitive hemopoietic organs, is made up of reticular cells, histiocytes, and macrophages functionally similar to those in the mesenchymal component of the liver.[1,14,15,27,35,36,48,60]

In tissue culture, connective tissue cells secrete free extracellular proteins immunologically identical with those of the species from which the cells were obtained.[103] Moreover, in tissue culture of unselected organs (without subculture of special cells strains), the connective tissue cells generally synthesize proteins and grow at a more prolific rate than the parenchymal cells.

The rate of isotope incorporation into intracellular proteins in tissue culture does not necessarily reflect the rate of free extracellular protein secretion from these cells under normal conditions. (Cf. item 7 of the above list indicating that liver cells secrete the bulk of the plasma proteins.)

Tissues which secrete significant quantities of free extracellular proteins are normally supplied with ducts into which the free extracellular proteins are secreted (along with water), e.g. pancreatic ducts, in the case of the entodermal cells of the pancreas; ducts named corresponding to the gland in the case of remaining compound tubular glands (mammary glands, salivary glands, prostate gland, etc.); lymph ducts (or lymphatics) in the case of lymph glands; and bile ducts in the case of the parenchymal cells of the liver. In the case of the mucosal cells lining the bronchial, alimentary, and genitourinary tracts, the free extracellular proteins, often recognized as mucoproteins, are secreted (along with water) into characteristic tubes or cavities.

Since no distinction is made between the functional role of hepatic mesenchymal and parenchymal cells, the perfusion experiments of Miller *et al.*[3-5] remain the primarily quoted authority for the popular conclusion that liver cells, presumably parenchymal cells, secrete the bulk of the plasma proteins, i.e. 100 percent of the albumin and 80 percent of remaining plasma proteins. These experiments were carried out by perfusing the portal vein of isolated rat livers with artificially pumped, mechanically oxygenated blood containing ^{14}C-labeled glycine, and analyzing for ^{14}C attached to free extracellular proteins in aliquots from the hepatic vein. In such experiments, the hepatic artery and hepatic efferent lymphatics were, of necessity, ligated and thus disregarded. To show that remaining body tissues secrete relatively little plasma protein, hepatectomized rat carcasses were perfused similarly via the distal thoracic–upper-abdominal aorta and aliquots sampled from the inferior vena cava which remained after removal of the liver. In the latter experiments, splenic venous and intestinal (portal) venous drainage into the perfusion circuit was eliminated by ligating the portal vein to remove the liver. Intestinal lymph and much of the carcass lymph drainage into the perfusion circuit was eliminated by ligating the systemic venous system proximal to the site of entry of the thoracic and cervical lymph ducts. Excluding the lungs and heart, by oxygenating artificially and pumping mechanically (with minimal pulse) in the anesthetized animal (whose spontaneous movements are minimal), undoubtedly the flow of lymph from any distal part was eliminated, thus eliminating contamination of the venous system by influx from lymphatics entering below the diaphragm. Moreover, as the bulk of the active red bone marrow (normally found in the axial skeleton, sternum, and ribs) drains via the vertebral and azygous system into the venous circulation above the diaphragm, a significant segment of red bone marrow drainage was disregarded, also. This effectively eliminated most of the definitive lymphoid and myeloid hemopoietic tissues from the perfusion circuit. It should therefore be easy to see why Miller *et al.* calculated that liver cells, irrespective of kind, synthesize the bulk of the plasma proteins and why the remaining tissues, including the lymphoid cells of the intestine, the organized lymphoid tissues elsewhere, the bone marrow, and remaining body tissues, synthesize relatively little.

A factor neglected in currently popular concepts of the cellular source of the plasma proteins is that in normal, healthy individuals, the blood and lymph plasma (and their proteins) do not originate primarily in the liver, but come from the water and food ingested, digested, and selectively absorbed via the intestine. Being independent of intestinal absorption and selection of substrate, tissue culture and perfusion systems supply environmental conditions somewhat different from those present in the internal milieu of the living individual.

With respect to assumptions based on clinical observations, individuals with cirrhosis or hepatitis are notoriously poor eaters, suffering from imbibition of alcohol to the exclusion of food, from profound anorexia, or both. Under such conditions, the liver must be expected to compensate plasma deficits in proteins and other substances along with, or at the expense of, other tissues (especially the lymphoid tissues which shrink more rapidly during starvation than remaining tissues in the body). When the liver fails to compensate, one sees not only hypoproteinemia with relative decrease in albumin but often a relative (compensatory) increase in protein synthesis in lymphoid tissues and bone marrow, as evidenced by relative increase in percentage of pyroninophilic cells.[110,111] Simutaneously, one may measure an increased turnover rate in some of the serum globulins, especially alpha-2 and beta globulin. Such findings can be explained relatively simply (after Reimann [102]) by considering that the liver plays an essential role in plasma protein metabolism, not by producing plasma proteins but by helping to maintain stability in circulating concentrations of small nitrogenous and other molecules from which tissue, blood cell, and plasma proteins are synthesized in diverse, distant tissues.

In conclusion, then, review of the selected clinical and experimental data, along with the embryological development and topographical anatomy of the liver, lends little to support the currently popular assumption that the liver, especially its parenchyme, produces the bulk of the plasma proteins in healthy, feeding individuals. Instead, the evidence indicates that the mesenchymal component of the liver functions as an auxiliary blood-forming organ, producing relatively large quantities of plasma and blood cells during vertebrate embryogenesis and continuing to produce plasma and some of its proteins (by clasmatosis) during adult life. The amount of plasma or plasma protein produced by the liver in comparison with that produced by the remaining definitive hemopietic organs (such as bone marrow, spleen, lymph nodes, and intestinal lymphoid tissue) is not clear from the experimental data at hand and remains to be ascertained with greater precision. It is probable that the relative quantities will be found to vary with the nutritional state. For example, during starvation, the liver (appended as it is to the intestine) can be expected to increase its relative rate of production by turning over cells, free extracellular proteins, fats, carbohydrates, and other simple compounds from other tissues to offset the relative lack of production from food absorbed via the intestine.

5. Tissues Supporting Parenchymal Cells and Dependent Primarily on Afferent Arterioles for Substrate

The peripheral connective tissues fall into the category of tissues supporting parenchymal cells and dependent primarily on afferent arteries for substrate. Like the reticular stroma of the marrow and spleen, they receive substrate primarily from afferent arterioles but differ from the former in that they do not support large numbers of developing blood cells and instead support various kinds of parenchymal cells of ectodermal, mesodermal, and entodermal derivation. The peripheral connective tissues differ from the reticular stroma of the intestine in that the supported parenchymal cells are not primarily concerned with absorption and hence are not a relatively direct source of substrate from food ingested. They differ, moreover, from the reticular stroma of the liver and lymph nodes in that afferent veins and afferent lymphatics are lacking. Therefore, afferent arterioles still remain the principal source of substrate.

Although the peripheral connective tissues, like the reticular stroma of the liver and the definitive hemopoietic organs, function as hemopoietic organs during embryogenesis and continue to give rise to relatively small numbers of histiocytes and macrophages during adult life,[1,14,15,34,36,55] their hemopoietic function becomes subordinate to their matrical function in support of adjacent parenchymal cells with increasing development of the latter and with the establishment of definitive blood circulation (see Chap. 24). During adult life, then, the peripheral connective tissues and the parenchymal cells supported become the focal point toward which the circulating output of the definitive hemopoietic organs is aimed and the focal point from which some, especially the regional lymph nodes, obtain feedback to govern or modify circulating output (see Chap. 18).

As emphasized by Maximow,[15,55] the reticular stroma of the definitive blood-forming organs and the connective tissue matrix supporting parenchymal cells are not only developmentally analogous but also endowed similarly with mesenchymal cells, especially reticular cells, fibroblasts, histiocytes, and macrophages. Moreover, pointing to secretory vacuole formation from some of the latter, he assumed the connective tissues in general to be sources of the plasma in the vessels.[15]

Currently, however, none of the connective tissues are considered to play an active or formative role in the production of lymph or plasma, or the free extracellular proteins found in either. Pursuant to the assumption (see above) that all the albumin and most of the globulins in the plasma are produced by the liver, the connective tissues, generally, and the peripheral connective tissues, specifically, are looked upon as supportive matrices through which diverse molecules from the circulating blood filter or pour to gain access to supported cells or to lymphatics.

Mechanistically (see Chap. 28), then, peripheral lymph is looked upon as an ultrafiltrate composed of water, salts, and free extracellular proteins which have filtered or leaked from the circulating blood through the semipermeable arteriovenous capillary endothelium and which have passed onward through intervening connective tissue to enter the lymphatics. While there is no question that diverse large and small molecules pass intact from the circulating blood to lymph, the currently popular "filtration" concept of lymph formation fails to explain what happens to those molecules, large and small, which fail to pass intact and which are reutilized for growth in the intervening connective tissue and in adjacent parenchymal cells.

Evidence that peripheral connective tissue and parenchymal cells continue to play an active role in hemopoiesis by contributing toward peripheral lymph formation may be summarized as follows.

Many of the diverse molecules which filter or pour through the endothelium of the peripheral arteriovenous capillaries are utilized for growth and function, both in the peripheral connective tissues and in the parenchymal cells which they support. To be numbered among the diverse molecules so utilized are proteins from the circulating blood, as evidenced by three facts. First, plasma proteins, irrespective of site of cellular origin, disappear from the circulating blood at finite rates varying with the kind of protein and are reutilized for growth in the tissues generally (as shown by Whpple).[112] Second, lipoproteins carried from the intestinal submucosa via the lymphatics to the general circulation are cleared in the periphery somewhere between the arteriovenous capillaries and the peripheral lymphatics. As a result, peripheral lymph normally is clear, whereas the blood plasma may be cloudy, particularly during the postprandial state. Third, similarly, somewhere between the peripheral arteriovenous capillaries and the peripheral lymphatics, a large proportion of the plasma proteins, particularly the globulins, disappear in a manner such that peripheral lymph carries a lower protein concentration and higher albumin: globulin ratio than arterial blood. The relatively low protein concentration and high albumin: globulin ratio in peripheral lymph can be explained by observations that the peripheral arteriovenous capillaries are relatively impermeable to free extracellular proteins, especially globulins. These findings can be explained, also, by the utilization of these proteins, especially the globulins, and production of relatively low molecular weight free extracellular proteins in the peripheral tissues. Since the peripheral connective tissue cells consist, to a large extent, of polymerized albuminoids [53] and are known to be quite soluble under certain physiologic situations, [53] one may suspect that upon dissolution, they may give rise to appreciable quantities of albuminoid proteins, along with free extracellular water.

As they grow through utilization of diverse molecules from the circulating blood, neither the peripheral connective tissue cells nor the parenchymal cells which they support are inert with respect to the production of free extracellular proteins. One need only transplant such cells between living individuals to ascertain that indeed they secrete extracellular proteins, known immunologically as antigens. The latter, in turn, sensitize cell populations in the regional and other lymphoid organs to produce additional free extracellular proteins known as antibodies and to produce cells recognizable as immunologically competent lymphocytes which normally proceed to agglutinate the antigens and destroy their living cellular sources (see Chap. 18).

One may confirm free extracellular protein production, also, by separating the parenchymal cells from connective tissue cells by artificial semipermeable membrances. If the pore sizes of the membranes are too small to allow passage or interchange of free extracellular proteins, neither the connective tissue cells nor the parenchymal cells will grow and differentiate normally in tissue culture. [113,114]

Moreover, it is common knowledge that some cells in certain

organs, such as the endocrine or ductless glands, secrete free extracellular proteins known as hormones into lymph and circulating blood. Similarly, other parenchymal cells, such as hepatic polygonal cells and muscle cells, under certain conditions (usually pathologic) may give rise to increased quantities of circulating free extracellular proteins recognizable biochemically as enzymes, e.g. transaminases. It should be interjected, however, that the quantities of free extracellular proteins excreted from parenchymal cells in the form of antigens, hormones, or enzymes are relatively small in comparison with the quantity of other free extracellular proteins normally present in the circulating body fluids. Whereas the former are measured primarily in terms of their profound catalytic effects on diverse tissues and can be measured directly only in terms of bioassay or fractions of milligrams percent, the latter can be measured simply in terms of grams percent. All such free extracellular proteins, nevertheless, can be expected to exert osmotic effects corresponding to molecular number and molecular size, regardless of cellular source or sources.

While the mesenchymal cells lining peripheral lymph capillaries, like those lining the sinusoids in the liver and in the definitive hemopoietic organs (see Chap. 24, D) are relatively permeable to proteins, in order to fill the peripheral lymphatics with lymph, sufficient proteins or other molecules, osmotically equivalent, must actually enter to attract water at the expense of surrounding tissues. Therefore, if some of the proteins and other molecules which filter or pour from the peripheral arteriovenous capillaries are utilized for growth and function in peripheral connective tissue and parenchymal cells, the latter must not only secrete sufficient osmotically equivalent molecules to replace those so utilized from leaking arteriovenous capillaries but also do so in sufficient excess to create a situation favorable to the osmotic attraction of water into the peripheral lymph capillaries.*

Endothelial cells having the capacity to filter, but apparently

---

* In the current symposia on lymphology, and for at least 100 years, heated, almost endless, discussion has centered on this point (see Chap. 28).

lacking the power to secrete a definitive product, only the peripheral connective tissue cells remain in a suitable position to do so. For the latter not only separate the arteriovenous from the lymph capillaries but also line portions of the latter uncovered by endothelium, particularly the peripheral tips. Here, like the primitive mesenchymal cells of the the developing embryo and their counterparts constituting the reticular stroma of the liver and of the definitive hemopoietic organs of the adult, the peripheral connective tissue cells occupy a position such that dissolution of their cytoplasm will not only contribute toward the production of plasma but also toward the production of liquid peripheral lymph capable of flowing and osmotically holding water to carry products from adjacent cells (along with unutilized molecules leaking from the adjacent, established arteriovenous capillaries,) toward the systemic circulation via peripheral lymphatics.

Thus one may envision the peripheral connective tissues not only as supportive matrices through which diverse molecules from the circulating blood diffuse to nourish growing parenchymal cells but also as segments of mesenchymal tissue actively involved in the production of peripheral lymph. Owing to the fact that the peripheral lymph itself is undoubtedly a mixture of products emanating from peripheral connective tissue cells, products emanating from the parenchymal cells which the connective tissue supports, and diverse molecules leaked from the peripheral arteriovenous capillaries, but unutilized by either of the former, it cannot be stated what percentage of the peripheral lymph or of its proteins are formed by the connective tissue cells alone. Moreover, owing to the fact that peripheral lymph flows to the regional nodes where diverse molecules may be removed while others are added (along with cells) to the centrally moving lymph stream, it cannot be stated with any degree of assurance how much plasma or how much plasma protein is generated normally in the peripheral connective tissues, as compared with that generated in the nodes. One may predict only that the peripheral connective tissues (like the reticular stroma of the blood froming organs) are significant sources of some of the water and relatively low molecular weight, osmotically important proteins in peripheral lymph. On the other hand, the organized lymphoid tissues are relatively important sources of some of the water and relatively high molecular weight, immunologically active, and nutritionally important proteins to be found in central lymph and in the circulating blood.

6. Summary and Conclusions

The circulating blood of the adult mammal is a mixture of formed elements and plasma produced in many hemopoietic tissues. While the exact tissue sources of specific types of formed elements are relatively obvious, the precise sources of specific plasma components are not. This is in part owing to the fact that although whole cells withstand the rigors of tissue fixation, soluble cytoplasmic droplets and free fluids do not. Also, the accurate identification of specific plasma components is obscured by the fact that hemic elements released from the bone marrow are promptly diluted into the contents of systemic veins; those released from the spleen are promptly diluted into the bloody contents of the portal system; those released from the mesenchymal component of the liver are promptly diluted into the contents of the venous sinusoids or into the hepatic lymphatics; and those released from the lymphatic tissues are diluted into centrally moving lymph containing elements of the blood plasma which have escaped from the arteriovenous capillaries.

Here, the afferent sources of molecular substrate necessary for specific hemopoietic activity in different hematopoietic tissues are analyzed. Whereas the bone marrow receives its entire molecular substrate supply via a relatively limited number of arterioles, the remaining hematopoietic tissues are more generously supplied with arterial blood or have additional sources from which molecular substrate may be assimilated. It would appear that whereas the marrow is oriented toward producing and maintaining the bulk of the formed elements in the blood, the remaining hematopoietic tissues are oriented toward producing and maintaining a very small volume of circulating lymphocytes and a large segment of the circulating plasma. Although rough qualitative estimates are made, the precise quantities and character of plasma proteins derived from each segment of the hematopoietic system remain to be clarified, correlated, and related further to those emanating from parenchymal cells throughout the body.

E. THE SIGNIFICANCE OF DISPARITIES IN VOLUME, FLOW, AND HISTOLOGIC DEVELOPMENT

While the hematopoietic tissues, the vessels, the blood, and the lymph can be looked upon as specific entities, basically they represent the means whereby molecular substrate can be transported through the massive vertebrate organism at rates and in quantities greater than these substances can move by the process of simple diffusion. In the 70 kg human, some 1200 gm of active marrow normally maintains 2.1 litres of erythrocytes to facilitate the transportation of oxygen within vessels serving almost all portions of the body. The remaining hematopoietic tissue, whose mass (700–1400 grams [32]) is roughly comparable to that of the bone marrow, normally maintains about 4 grams of lymphocytes and a (presumptively) great share of the 3.1 liters of plasma in the vascular system. The plasma facilitates the transportation of water, amino acids, fats, proteins, and many other substances. The circulating lymphocytes, possessing the power of independent motility, may carry their constituent proteins, nucleic acids, etc., onward into the tissues at rates more rapid than some of these substances can move by the process of diffusion alone. As suggested definitively by Kelsall and Crabb,[105] these circulating lymphocytes may then function as trephocytes, releasing their high-molecular-weight proteins and nucleic acids to nourish the various tissues which they ultimately invade.

In the nutritional sense, if all suggestions are correct, one may consider the relatively immobile, larger lymphocytes and other mononuclear cells within hematopoietic tissues as cells designed to facilitate the transport of diverse small and large molecules through their role in plasma formation, whereas the more mobile, smaller circulating lymphocytes and monocytes may be looked upon as cells admirably designed to speed the transport of the largest, least-diffusible molecules directly to the tissues.

It is developmentally significant to note that the 5.2 liters of whole blood normally maintained within the vascular system of the 70 kg. human is insufficient to match the relatively large volume capacity attained by the vascular system during its growth. This disparity is reflected acutely in the state of clinical shock which develops when too many vascular channels open simultaneously. Normally, in the compensated state, this disparity is reflected in the concerted activity of the vessels, thoroughfares, capillaries, and sinusoids—with the vessels and thoroughfares carrying a segment of the total volume constantly, while capillaries and sinusoids carry the remaining volume intermittently. This disparity between volume and volume capacity and its reflection in disparate flow and development in the different types of circulatory channels is of fundamental importance not only to the logic of this analysis but also to a logical concept of the potentialities for continued growth and modification within the hemic and vascular systems. To illustrate: in the distal portions of the thoroughfare arteriovenous channels where the share of flow is of a lower order than that in the vessels, the muscular tunics and innervation thin out to become almost rudimentary.[40-44] Here the thoroughfares resemble the capillaries in structure. In the true capillaries where the share of flow is of an even lower order, a few of the lining cells have been held to differ from common vascular endothelial cells in that they retain the capacity for differentiation into hemic cells,[51-52,58] and they are observed to be relatively permeable to proteins.[56,64] Here the capillaries bear a functional resemblance to the sinusoids. In the sinusoids where the share of flow is presumably of the lowest order, a significant segment of the lining tissue resembles undifferentiated mesenchyme in that the constituent units (nucleocytoplasmic territories[50]) lack cellular boundaries, reticular fibrils, and specific cytoplasmic structures such as granules, inclusions, or ingested materials, and remain capable of differentiation into blood cells, histiocytes, fibroblasts, and endothelial cells.[31,35,36,48,55,59-61] Here the sinusoids resemble the demarcating blood puddles in the mesenchyme of the early embryo before blood flow has actually commenced.

These examples of disparate flow in conjunction with dis-

parate development within the different types of channels suggest that each specialized type of channel has differentiated out
of the more primitive as a direct result of an increasing share of
flow (as suggested 75 years ago by Thoma [106]) and that just as
the cardiovascular system is never completely filled and flow,
consequently, never becomes constant in some portions of the
system, some portions of the system never complete their differentiation. This relative lack of differentiation is reflected not
only in the comparative structure of the existing vessels, thoroughfares, capillaries, sinusoids, and reticulum but also in the capacity
of these structures for modification in compliance with changing
conditions. Such capacities may include the capacity for progressive transformations, such as the transformation of the reticulum
into sinusoids,[31,60] of sinusoids into capillaries,[59] and of capillaries
into thoroughfares and vessels,[107] in addition to the capacity for
reproduction of these structures in kind.[108] They may also include
the capacity for retrogressive transformation, such as the resumption of marrow-like activity within the sinusoidal reticulum of the
liver [61,87] and within the reticular connective tissues supporting
extramedullary capillaries.[51,52,87,109]

Chapter 26

SUMMARY

UTILIZING DIFFUSIBLE MOLECULAR substrate, first directly from the yolk sac entoderm and later from vessels in varying stages of organization, the embryonal mesenchyme of each body area undergoes hypertrophy, differentiation, and dissolution to create isolated puddles of whole blood or lymph. In each area, the puddles subsequently coalesce and then circulation actually commences as a result of rhythmic cardiac or skeletal muscular contractions. At this time, the mesenchyme differentiates further into endothelial tubes whose degree of differentiation appears proportional to the flow rate locally established. In areas where flow remains inconstant, as in the sinusoids of the definitive hematopoietic organs, the mesenchyme gives rise to reticuloendothelium, a tissue less differentiated, more permeable, and possessing a higher order of phagocytic activity than the common vascular endothelium lining capillaries and vessels. It is suggested that during adult life, the whole blood and lymph continue to arise in the reticulum of various hemopoietic organs just as they do in the diffuse mesenchyme of the embryo; that is by hypertrophy of the mesenchymal reticular matrix, by differentiation of individual blood cells, and by dissolution of the matrix. Because the matrix is essentially a gel made up of water and highly polymerized, low-molecular-weight proteins, it is suggested that its dissolution will yield plasma consisting of water and low-molecular-weight, osmotically important proteins. Additional plasma, rich in high-molecular-weight proteins, may arise by dissolution of cytoplasmic droplets (hyaline bodies) shed from many mesenchymally derived mononuclear cells such as histiocytes, monocytes, plasma cells and lymphocytes. It is stressed that dissolution of the gelatinous reticular matrix will not only free the formed elements and their various cytoplasmic products from a fixed tissue position but also will supply a sol

15. Maximow, A.: Relation of blood cells to connective tissues and endothelium. *Physiol Rev, 4*:533–563, 1924.

16. Stockard, C. R.: The origin of blood and vascular endothelium in embryos without a circulation of the blood and in the normal embryo. *Amer J Anat, 18*:227–327, 1915.

17. Clark, E. R.: Studies on the growth of blood vessels in the tail of the frog larva—by observation and experiment on the living animal. *Amer J Anat, 23*:37–89, 1918.

18. Gilmour, J. R.: Normal haemopoiesis in intrauterine and neonatal life. *J Path Bact, 52*:25–55, 1941.

19. Sabin, F. R.: *The Origin and Development of the Lymphatic System.* Baltimore, John Hopkins Press, 1913.

20. Huntington, G. S.: The development of the mammalian jugular lymph sac, of the tributary primitive ulnar lymphatic and of the thoracic ducts from the viewpoint of recent investigations of vertebrate lymphatic ontogeny, together with a consideration of the genetic relations of lymphatic and haemal vascular channels in embryos of amniotes. *Amer J Anat, 16*:259–316, 1914.

21. McClure, C. F. W.: The development of the lymphatic system in the light of more recent investigation in the field of vasculogenesis. *Anat Rec, 9*:563–579, 1915.

22. Kampmeier, O. F.: Ursprung und Engwicklungsgeschichte des Ductus thoracicus nebst Saccus lymphaticus jugularis und Cysterna chyli beim Menschen. *Morphol Jahrb, 67*:157–234, 1931. (Göppert Festschrift II).

23. Zimmerman, A. A.: *Origin and Development of the Lymphatic System in Opossum.* Urbana, University of Illinois Press, 1940.

24. Danchakoff, V.: Equivalence of different hematopoietic anlages. *Amer J Anat, 24*:127–189, 1918.

25. Hammond, W. S.: On the origin of the cells lining the liver sinusoids in the cat and rat. *Amer J Anat, 65*:199–228, 1939.

26. Bloch, E. H.: The *in vivo* microscopic anatomy and physiology of the liver as determined with the quartz rod method of transillumination. *Angiology, 6*:340–349, 1955.

27. Mann, J. D. and Higgins, C. M.: The system of fixed histiocytes in the liver. In Downey, H. (Ed.): *Handbook of Hematology.* New York, Hoeber, 1938, vol. 2, pp. 1375–1426.

28. Shields, J. W.: On the relationship between growing blood cells and blood vessels. *Acta Haematol, 24*:319–329, 1960.

29. Downey, H. and Weidenreich, F.: Ueber die Bildung der Lymphocyten in Lymphdrüsen und Milz. *Arch Mikr Anat Entwicklungsgesch, 80*:306–395, 1912.

30. Downey, H.: On the development of lymphocytes in lymph nodes and spleen. Transactions. *Minn Path Soc, 1*:91–102, 1912.

31. Downey, H.: The structure and origin of the lymph sinuses of mammalian lymph nodes and their relations to endothelium and reticulum. *Haematologica, 3*:431–468, 1922.

32. Drinker, C. K. and Yoffey, J. M.: *Lymphatics, Lymph and Lymphoid tissue.* Cambridge, Harvard University Press, 1941.

33. Thiel, G. and Downey, H.: The development of the mammalian spleen with special reference to its hematopoietic activity. *Amer J Anat, 28*:279–333, 1921.

34. Bloom, W.: Lymphatic tissue, lymphatic organs. In Downey, H. (Ed.): *Handbook of Hematology.* New York, Hoeber, 1938, vol. 2, pp. 1427–1468.

35. Aschoff, L.: Das reticulo-endotheliale system. Ergeln Inn Med. *Kinderheilk, 26*:1–119, 1924. (Also in *Lectures on Pathology.* New York, Paul B. Hoeber, 1924, pp. 1–33.)

36. Jaffé, R. H.: The reticulo-endothelial System. In Downey, H. (Ed.): *Handbook of Hematology.* New York, Hoeber, 1938, vol. 2, pp. 937–1272.

37. Brånemark, I.: Experimental investigation of microcirculation in bone marrow. *Angiology, 12*:293–305, 1961.

38. Doan, C. A.: Bone marrow. Normal and pathologic physiology with special reference to diseases involving the cells of the blood. In Downey, H. (Ed.): *Handbook of Hematology.* New York, Hoeber, 1938, vol. 3, pp. 1839–1962.

39. Ehrich, W. E.: The role of the lymphocyte in the circulation of lymph. *Ann N Y Acad Sci, 46*:823–857, 1946.

40. Krogh, A.: *The Anatomy and Physiology of Capillaries.* New Haven, Yale University Press, 1929.

41. Zweifach, B. W.: The structure and reactions of the small blood vessels in amphibia. *Amer J Anat, 60*:473–514, 1937.

42. Zweifach, B. W.: The character and distribution of the blood capillaries. *Anat Rec, 73*:475–495, 1939.

43. Chambers, R. and Zweifach, B. W.: Functional activity of the blood capillary bed, with special reference to visceral tissue. *Ann N Y Acad Sci, 46*:683–695, 1946.

44. Zweifach, B. W.: General principles governing the behaviour of the microcirculation. *Amer J Med, 23*:684–696, 1957.

45. Knisely, M. H.: Microscopic observations of the circulatory system of living unstimulated mammalian spleens. *Anat Rec, 65*:23–50, 1936.

46. MacKenzie, D. W., Whipple, A. O., and Wintersteiner, M. P.: Studies on microscopic anatomy and physiology of living transilluminated mammalian spleens. *Amer J Anat, 68*:397–456, 1941.

47. Parpart, A. K., Whipple, A. O., and Chang, J. J.: The microcirculation of the spleen of the mouse. *Angiology, 6*:350–368, 1955.

48. Klemperer, P.: The spleen. In Downey, H. (Ed.) : *Handbook of Hematology.* New York, Hoeber, 1938, vol. 3, pp. 1587–1754.
49. Hueck, W.: Ueber das Mesenchyme. *Beitr Path Anat, 66*:330–374, 1920.
50. Bennett, H. S., Luft, J. H., and Hampton, J. C.: Morphological classifications of vertebrate blood capillaries. *Amer J Physiol, 196*:381–390, 1959.
51. Marchand, F.: Ueber die Bedeutung der sogenannten grosskernigen Wanderzellen sitzunsb. *Ges Beford Ges Naturw, 6*:105, 1897.
52. Herzog, G.: Uber die bedeutugun der gafässwandzellen in der pathologie *Klin Wschr, 2*:684–689, 1923.
53. Gersh, I., and Catchpole, H. H.: The organization of ground substance and basement membrane and its significance in tissue injury, and growth. *Amer J Anat, 85*:457–523, 1949.
54. Folkow, B.: Nervous control in blood vessels. *Physiol Rev, 35*:629–663, 1955.
55. Maximow, A. A.: Morphology of the mesenchymal reactions. *Arch Path Lab Med, 4*:557–606, 1927.
56. Zweifach, B. W.: Pathophysiology of the blood vascular barrier. *Angiology, 13*:345–355, 1962.
57. Stchelkounoff, S. I.: L'intima des petites artères et des veins et le mésenchyme vasculaire. *Arch Anat Micr, 32*:139–194, 1936.
58. McJunkin, F.: The origin of the phagocytic mononuclear cells of the peripheral blood. *Amer J Anat, 25*:27, 1919.
59. McJunkin, F.: Transformation of sinusoidal endothelium into the ordinary capillary type. *Amer J Path, 7*:9–12, 1931.
60. Klemperer, P.: The relationship of the reticulum to diseases of the hematopoietic system. In: Contribution to the medical sciences in honor of Doctor Emanuel Libman by his pupils, friends, and colleagues. New York, International Press, 1932, pp. 655–672.
61. Bloom, W.: Myelepoietic potency of fixed cells of the rabbit liver. *Libman Anniv. Vols. (II),* pp. 199–207, 1932.
62. Chambers, R. and Zweifach, B. W.: Capillary endothelial cement in relation to permeability. *J Cell Comp Physiol, 15*:255–272, 1940.
63. Kiyono, K.: *Die vitale Karminspeicherung.* Jena, Fischer, 1914.
64. Pappenheimer, J. R.: Passage of molecules through capillary walls. *Physiol Rev, 33*:387–423, 1953.
65. Fawcett, D. W.: The fine structure of capillaries, arterioles, and small arteries in the microcirculation. In Reynolds, S. R. M. and Zweifach, B. W. (Eds.) : *The Microcirculation.* Urbana, University of Illinois Press, 1959, pp. 1–27.
66. Renkin, E. M.: Capillary permeability and transcapillary exchange in relation to molecular size. In Reynolds, S. R. M. and Zweifach, B. W. (Eds.) : *The Microcirculation.* Urbana, University of Illinois Press, 1959, pp. 28–46.

67. Whipple, A. O., Parpart, A. K., and Chang, J. J.: A study of the circulation of the blood in the spleen of the living mouse. *Ann. Surg.,* *140*:266–269, 1954.

68. Copenhaver, W. M.: Heart, blood vessels, blood, and entodermal derivatives. In Willier, B. H., Weiss, P. A., and Hamburger, V. (Eds.) : *Analysis of Development.* Philadelphia, Saunders, 1955, pp. 440–461.

69. Torrey, T. W.: *Morphogenesis of the Vertebrates.* New York, John Wiley, 1962, 600 pp.

70. Isaacs, R.: The physiological histology of bone marrow: The mechanism of the development of blood cells and their liberation into the peripheral circulation. *Folia Haemat, 40*:395–405, 1930.

71. Bloom, W.: Lymphocytes and monocytes: theories of hematepoiesis. In Downey, H. (Ed.) : *Handbook of Hematology.* New York, Hoeber, 1938, pp. 375–435 and 1551–1585.

72. Downey, H.: The origin of blood platelets. *Folia Haemat, 15* (1) :25–58, 1913.

73. Shields, J. W.: On the function of lymphoid tissue. *Proceedings of the IX Congress of the International Society of Hematology, 3*:621–629, 1964.

74. White, A. and Dougherty, T. F.: The role of lymphocytes in normal and immune globulin production and the mode of release of globulin from lymphocytes. *Ann N Y Acad Sci, 46*:859–882, 1942.

75. White, A.: Influence of endocrine secretions on the structure and function of lymphoid tissue. In *Harvey Lectures.* Springfield. Thomas, 1950, pp. 43–70.

76. Landis, E. M.: Capillary permeability and the factors affecting the composition of capillary filtrate. *Ann N Y Acad Sci, 46*:713–731, 1946.

77. Rich, A. R., Lewis, M. R., and Wintrobe, M. M.: The activity of the lymphocytes in the body's reaction to foreign protein as established by the identification of the acute splenic tumor cell. *Bull. Johns Hopkins Hosp., 65*:311–327, 1939.

78. Fagraeus, A. L.: Antibody production in relation to the development of plasma cells. *Acta Med Scand* (supp) *204,* 1948.

79. Gunderson, C. H., Juras, D., La Via, M. F., and Wissler, R. W.: Antibody formation in the rat spleen. *JAMA, 108*:1038–1047, 1962.

80. Hofmeister, F.: Untersuchungen uber Resorption und Assimilation der Nahrstoffe. *Arch Exp Path Pharmkol, 19*:1–33, 1885.

81. Harris, I. N. and Harris, S.: Histochemical changes in lymphocytes during production of antibodies in lymph nodes of rabbits. *J Exp Med, 90*:169–179, 1949.

82. Ehrich, W. E., Drabkin, D. L., and Furman, C. L.: Nucleic acids and the production of antibody by plasma cells. *J. Exp Med, 90*:157–167, 1949.

83. Bessis, M. C. and Breton-Gorius, J.: Ferritin and ferruginous micelles in normal erythroblasts and hypochromic hypersideremic anemias. *Blood, 14*:423–432, 1959.

84. Sundberg, R. D.: Lymphocytes: Origin, structure, and inter-relationships. In Rebuck, J. W. (Ed.) : *The Lymphocyte and Lymphocytic Tissue.* New York, Hoeber, 1960, pp. 1–21.

85. Ranvier, L.: Des clasmatocytes. *Compt Rend Acad Sci, 110*:165–189, 1890.

86. Sabin, F. R.: Cellular reactions to a dye-protein with a concept of the mechanism of antibody formation. *J Exp Med, 70*:67–81, 1939.

87. Lang, F. J.: Myeloid metaplasia. In Downey, H. (Ed.) : *Handbook of Hematology.* New York, Hoeber, 1938, vol 3, pp. 2103–2144.

88. Grant, J. L. and Smith, B.: Bone marrow gas tensions, bone marrow blood flow and erythropoiesis in man. *Ann. Int. Med., 58*:801–809, 1963.

89. Bierman, H. R., Kelly, K. H., White, L. P., Corblentz, A. and Fisher, A.: Transhepatic venous catheterization and venography. *JAMA, 158*:1331–1334, 1955.

90. Trowell, O. A.: Experiments on lymph nodes cultured *in vitro. Ann N Y Acad Sci, 59*:1066–1069, 1955.

91. Barcroft, J.: Alterations in the volume of the normal spleen and their significance. *Amer J Med Sci, 179*:1–10, 1930.

92. Crosby, W. H.: Normal functions of the spleen relative to red blood cells. *Blood, 14*:399–408, 1959.

93. Doan, C. A.: Hypersplenism. *Bull N Y Acad Med, 25*:625–650, 1949.

94. Brachet, J.: The localization and the role of ribonucleic acid in the cell. *Ann N Y Acad Sci, 50*:861–869, 1950.

95. McMaster, P. D.: Sites of antibody formation. In Pappenheimer, A. M. (Ed.) : The nature and significance of the antibody response. New York, Columbia University Press, 1953, pp. 13–45.

96. Ivy, A. C.: Gastrointestinal changes in the rat on realimentation. *Amer J Physiol, 195*:216–220, 1958.

97. Cantarow, A. and Trumper, M.: Clinical biochemistry. Philadelphia, Saunders, 1955.

98. Wintrobe, M. M.: Relation of disease of the liver to anemia. *Arch Int Med, 57*:289–306, 1936.

99. White, A.: *Principles of Biochemistry.* New York, McGraw-Hill, 1954.

100. Seligson, D.: Biochemical considerations of the liver. In Schiff, L. (Ed.) : *Disease of the Liver.* Philadelphia, Lippincott, 1956, pp. 50–91.

101. Reimann, H. A., Medes, G. and Fisher, L. The origin of blood proteins. *Folia Haematol, 53*:187–202, 1934.

102. Peters, T. and Anfnsen, C. B.: Net production of serum albumin by liver slices. *J. Biol. Chem., 186*:805–813, 1950.

103. Landsteiner, K. and Parker, R. C.: Serologic tests for homologous serum proteins in tissue cultures maintained on a foreign medium. *J Exp Med, 71*:231–236, 1940.

104. Carnot, P. and Gruzewska, Z.: L'elimination des nucleoproteides par la bile. *Compt Rend Soc Biol, 99*:598–601, 1928.

105. Kelsall, M. A. and Crabb, E. D.: *Lymphocytes and Mast Cells.* Baltimore, Williams and Wilkins, 1959.

106. Thoma, R.: Untersuchungen Uber die Histiogenese und Histomechanik des Gefass systems. Stuttgart, 1893.

107. Christiansen, G. E. and Bacon, R. L.: Direct observations of developing microcirculatory patterns in the posterior limb buds of fetal mice. *Angiology 12*:517, 1961.

108. Clark, E. R. and Clark, E. L.: Observations of living mammalian lymphatic capillaries—their relation to blood vessels. *Amer J Anat, 60*:253–298, 1937.

109. Möllendorf, W. and Möllendorf, M.: Das Fibrocytennetz im lockeren bindegewebe; sein wandlungsfäkigkeit und anteilnahme am Stoffwechsel. *Z Zellforsch, 3*:503–614, 1926.

110. Glagov, S., Kent, G., and Popper, H.: Relation of splenic and lymph node changes to hypergolbulinemia in cirrhosis. *Arch Path, 67*:9–18, 1959.

111. Alperin, P. M., Bumagina, T. K., Zherebtsov, L. A., Zamchy, A. A., and Rodina, R. I.: Bone marrow reticulo-plasmacytic reaction and blood proteins in patients with cirrhosis of the liver. *Probl Gemat 15*: 20–27, 1970.

112. Whipple, G. H.: *The Dynamic Equilibrium of Body Proteins.* Springfield, Thomas, 1956.

113. Grobstein, C.: Tissue interaction in the morphogenesis of mouse embryonic rudiments in vitro. In Rudnick, D. (Ed.): *Aspects of Synthesis and Order in Growth.* Princeton, Princeton University Press, p. 954.

114. Grobstein, C.: Cytodifferentiation and its controls. *Science, 143*:643–650, 1964.

Section 4

CONCEPTS NEW AND OLD

Chapter 27

AN INTEGRATED TROPHIC SYSTEM

A FUNDAMENTAL FUNCTION OF mesenchymal derivatives, such as lymphocytes, other mononuclear cells, lymph,
blood, lymph and blood vessesls, and connective tissues, is to
feed other cells in the body. In support of this thesis, it is shown
how the mononuclear cells derived from mesenchyme perform
their trophic functions by donating protoplasmic substance to
one another, into the vascular system, and ultimately to other
cells in the body. Particularly stressed is where they normally
obtain the substrate to synthesize the protoplasm which they subsequently donate. It is shown how relative lack of mononuclear
donors, especially small lymphocytes, results in atrophy or dis-
orderly growth in other body cells and in failure of the individual
to thrive. How the various mesenchymal derivatives develop together to constitute an integrated trophic system can be summarized in simple concept.

In embryos, the mesenchyme, or (Greek) "middle juice," is a
definitive tissue which gives matrical support and mediates the
transport of nourishment between cells of the body. Throughout
embryogenesis and phylogenesis, as the body grows by increase
in number and variety of component cells, the mesenchyme
grows correspondingly to produce increasing numbers and varieties of definitive cells, all destined to cooperate in carrying out
this supportive and nutritive function. As growth and differentiation proceed, the supportive function is borne out by mesenchymal derivatives of increasing solidarity, such as fibroblasts,
chondroblasts, and osteoblasts, whereas the nutritive function is
carried out by mesenchymal derivatives capable of giving rise to
or entering into a juicy or liquid medium, such as reticular cells,
histiocytes, macrophages, and various kinds of formed elements
(erythrocytes, platelets, and leucocytes). Just as increasing solidarity of the former enhances their supportive function, the

ability to enter into a fluid state enhances the nutritive function of the latter. This is due to the fact that fluids are capable of *flowing* to carry diverse dissolved molecules or suspended formed elements from one part of the body to another at rates much faster than either could move through solid tissues by diffusion or by virtue of their capacity for independent motility.

Essentially a gelatinous matrix, sometimes called ground substance, the mesenchyme commences relatively rapid growth and differentiation beneath the yolk sac entoderm which it grows to support and from which it commences to receive substrate necessary for growth and differentiation. As it grows outward from the yolk sac entoderm, portions dissolve to create puddles of fluid, called plasma. As differentiation proceeds, increasing numbers of mesenchymal derivatives add to this fluid by shedding cytoplasmic portions which dissolve, by releasing cytoplasmic portions which remain microscopically visible, or by entering in the form of intact cells of various morphologic description, all being released by dissolution of the matrix to become suspended in the fluid derived therefrom. As composites differentiated in this manner, the body fluids, blood and lymph, are created in separate isolated puddles whose contents are destined to circulate and thereby transport various substances to other tissues.

Transport actually commences when separtate puddles coalesce and their contents are impelled to flow under the impetus generated by rhythmic muscular contractions in neighboring tissues. Under this impetus which becomes translated into hydrostatic pressure, some of the mesenchyme flattens under intraluminal pressure to become the endothelium of definitive conduits, known as vessels. The remaining mesenchyme, meanwhile, continues differentiation in matrical support of the endothelium on the one hand, and of all remaining tissue cells on the other. The fluid-filled, mesenchyme-encased, endothelium-lined vessels, then, continue growth in girth and length by replication of endothelial cells, along with further growth and differentiation of supporting mesenchymal and muscular layers. Such differentiations are proportional to the velocity of flow established.

In organisms possessing mediastinal hearts,* the composite resulting from these successive differentiations is a fluid-filled vascular system made up of two separately derived, but complementary components. The first is a blood vascular system wherein flow is impelled directly and rapidly by the contractile activity of heart muscle and which is filled (a) with relatively large quantities of formed elements produced in myeloid organs (wherein blood flow remains inconstant in channels known as sinusoids; see Sect. 3), (b) with small molecules, such as water, oxygen, carbon dioxide, and urea, which diffuse quite freely from surrounding, adjacent tissues, and (c) with lymph emanating from the peripheral tissues and the organized lymphoid tissues (such as nodes) which intervene, this lymph being conveyed to the great veins of the lower neck by paired cervical and thoracic lymph ducts. The second component is a lymph vascular system wherein flow is impelled relatively slowly and intermittently by muscle contractions in tissues other than the mediastinal heart, and which is filled (a) with large and small molecules filtering from the blood vascular system, along with large and small molecules absorbed through or excreted from cells outside of the vascular system and (b) with relatively large molecules and cells produced in specialized lymphoid organs through reutilization of many of the former for growth. Although each of these systems takes its origin quite analogously but separately from growing, dissolving, differentiating mesenchyme located adjacent to definitive sources of molecular substrate, the differential development of the lymphatic system is predicated upon the prior development of flow in and filtration of molecular substrate, especially oxygen, from the blood vascular system.

Early in the embryogenesis of placentates which possess relatively little yolk but ultimately require relatively large quantities of circulating body fluids to fill extensive vascular systems, the production of these fluids shifts quite early from the yolk sac and general body mesenchyme to the mesenchymal component

---

* In lower forms of animal life which lack hearts, the body fluids circulate in relatively slow and haphazard fashion, are largely contained within mesenchymal spaces unlined by definitive endothelium, and lack hemoglobin pigment bound to cells. As a result, the circulating body fluids resemble lymph, rather than blood.

of the liver. Having used its relatively small supply of yolk to produce a complex fluid which can flow, a primitive heart to impel flow, and primitive vessels to conduct flowing fluids, the developing mammalian embryo becomes prepared upon nidation to circulate substrate absorbed via the placenta through the vitelline circulation to the liver.

The placental circulation, as an appendage and direct outgrowth from the primitive vessels developed earlier beneath the yolk sac entoderm, becomes the main pathway of absorption of substrate essential to growth, while the mesenchymal component of the liver, receiving substrate from the waning yolk sac entoderm and the waxing placenta, becomes the principal hemopoietic organ during the midportion of embryonal life. However, later in gestation as circulation becomes increasingly developed and rapid, as the placenta becomes larger and capable of absorbing increasing quantities of oxygen, and an increasing arteriovenous oxygen difference becomes established, the fetus must prepare to survive by breathing air and eating food. Correspondingly, myelopoiesis gradually recedes from the mesenchymal component of the liver to an environment of relatively low oxygen tension in the bone marrow, while lymphopoiesis evolutes in a periarterial environment of relatively high oxygen tension in the scattered lymphoid organs. The myeloid derivatives of mesenchyme remain largely concerned with the production of red cells which carry oxygen via the vascular system to the tissues. The lymphoid derivatives meanwhile remain largely concerned (as outlined in Sects. 1 and 3) with the production of lymph which flows centrally to constitute milky plasma in circulating whole blood. From the red cells and plasma flowing in arterial blood are derived relatively constant supplies of oxygen and food to sustain growth and function in all tissues. For it is toward the latter that the circulating output of the hemopoietic organs, myeloid and lymphoid, is ultimately aimed; and it is primarily in arterial blood that one sees relative constancy in the concentration of all blood constituents (after the mixing of venous blood and central lymph has taken place in the pulmonary circuit).

By the time of birth in most higher mammalian orders the

myeloid differentiation of mesenchyme has achieved adult configuration, erythropoiesis being confined to the marrow cavities. On the other hand, the lymphoid differentiation of mesenchyme does not achieve adult configuration for some time after placental connections are severed and the newborn has actually started breathing air and absorbing all subsequent nourishment via the intestine. The latter events signal the onset of thymic involution, and the consequent rapid growth of all remaining lymphoid organs, particularly the lymphoid tissue of the intestine (see Sect. 2). The lymphoid derivatives of mesenchyme, then, commence to show characteristic specialization to definitive trophic functions which can be outlined as follows.

The intestinal lymphoid tissue becomes specialized to produce central lymph from food absorbed via the intestinal mucosa each time a meal is absorbed.

The spleen becomes specialized to selectively break down, reutilize, store and release arterial blood components (especially cells and free extracellular proteins) emanating from all hemopoietic organs, including the intestinal lymphoid tissue, marrow, thymus, and nodes—all of which ultimately pour their circulating products into the central venous circulation prior to mixing in the pulmonary circuit.

The nodes become specialized to selectively break down, reutilize, store, and release components (especially proteins) of peripheral lymph which flows in from the tissues *to the end that these components can be reutilized for immunologic, as well as trophic purposes*, upon leaving via central lymph.

The thymus becomes specialized to produce, store, and release relatively large quantities of lymphocytes (or their disintegration products), as well as an entodermal hormone which accelerates their reutilization for lymphopoiesis in all the aforementioned definitive lymphoid organs.

Thus demarcated is a definitive hemopoietic system consisting of myeloid and lymphoid components which cooperate in the continued production of *whole blood* from food absorbed by the intestine, from the combined circulating output of diverse hemopoietic organs, and from molecules excreted from peripheral tissues which the mesenchyme has thus differentiated to serve.

Needless to say, the concept would be incomplete without indicating the role of the liver which, having ostensibly ceased production of circulating blood cells, is not ordinarily defined as a hemopoietic organ in adult mammals. Developing in the transverse septal mesenchyme out of the evaginating entoderm of the primitive gut such that it receives the entire portal effluent from the spleen and small intestine, as well as a relatively small share of the body's arterial blood, the liver resides in an appropriate position to break down, reutilize, store, and reconstitute the molecular constituents of circulating cells, free extracellular proteins and many smaller molecules circulated in from all the aforementioned sources. The products of the concerted activity of the hepatic mesenchymal (principally histiocytic) and parenchymal cells ultimately are excreted via bile into the small intestine, or released back into the vascular system to be available for hemopoiesis elsewhere (as outlined in Chap. 25, Sect. 4). No wonder the clinical assessment of liver function is difficult!

With respect to the integrated trophic function of individual types of cells which develop out of the mesenchyme, one may conceive of the various mononuclear lymphoid cells as donors of protoplasm which is donated in different ways, but ultimately reutilized as food in other cells. As stationary cells growing in the hemopoietic organs and liver, all donate protoplasm to create plasma. One may conceive of the plasma, then, as a milky fluid having many sources contributing singly and together toward the transport of formed elements and the transport of molecules essential to the nutrition of many tissues. The cytoplasm of the reticular cells, in addition, forms the matrix or *ground substance* in which all hemopoietic and parenchymal cells are embedded and from which the latter imbibe their sustenance while growing. Called the *reticular connective tissue* or *reticulum* during adult life, this *stroma* constitutes a *matrix* through which all incoming and outgoing molecules must diffuse or be carried from all growing cells, parenchymal and hemopoietic. As such it remains mesenchyme in purest form, and the very heart of the internal milieu described in physiologic terms by Claude Bernard. The remaining mononuclear cells, such as histiocytes, macrophages, monocytes, plasmacytes and lymphocytes, which develop out of the reticulum can be perceived as having augmentary trophic functions as outlined throughout the fore text (especially pp. 74-81) —some digesting visible macromolecules before shedding cytoplasm, some shedding cytoplasm without evidence of phagocytic activity, and others donating residual protoplasm (chiefly nucleoplasm) after migration from their sites of origin in the hemopoietic organs. Lymphocytes being the most numerous and common of mononuclear cells within (see Fig. 1b) and outside of the hemopoietic organs during adult life, they must be calculated to be most important protoplasmic donors. More obvious and well known, of course, is the trophic role of erythrocytes which donate oxygen to the tissues. Less obvious, perhaps, is the trophic role of the polymorphonuclear leucocytes which originate and migrate from the marrow to engulf and digest endogenous and foreign material, so that upon their death and dissolution as "pus" cells, all may be reutilized again. Opsonins and agglutinins produced by some of the mononuclear cells appear to enhance such activities on the part of the polymorphonuclear leucocytes.

Of course, the immunologic role of various mesenchymal derivatives, such as lymphocytes, plasmacytes, macrophages and polymorphonuclear leucocytes, has attracted great attention in recent years. Although not emphasized recently, it is an old concept that certain mesenchymal cells, such as histiocytes and macrophages, prepare noxious material (endogenous and foreign) as food for other cells in the host. Such activity is the literal meaning of opsonization. Extending this older concept, one may envision multiple kinds of cells being involved (as outlined in Sects. 2 and 3). For instance (and in order as a function of time), the histiocytes and macrophages perform initial digestion of noxious foreign or endogenous macromolecules, and shed the digested products by clasmatosis. The reticular precursors of plasmacytes reutilize some of the shed cytoplasm, as well as substrate from other sources, to produce plasmacytes which shed immunoglobulins and cytoplasmic RNA. The immunoglobulins may serve as circulating opsonins, while some of the RNA may be reutilized to transcribe additional codes on the DNA of lymphocyte pre-

cursors in the reticulum. Lymphocytes differentiating from the
latter, while growing within the reticulum, may shed additional
cytoplasm, some of whose dissolutionary products may be recognized as plasma and some of which may be recognized as very
specific agglutinins. That which remains of the lymphocytes after
shedding cytoplasm, i.e. small cytoplasm-poor lymphocytes, ultimately migrate into the circulation to give up their remaining
substance to other cells directly, or to lyse living sources of
obnoxious foreign or endogenous proteins. In the latter case
these living sources are reduced into simple substrate which can
be reutilized as palatable food for various kinds of cells in the
host. Such a concept not only takes into account the trophic function of certain cells toward others, but also the recognition
processes essential to the consummation of successful immunologic
reactions.

Obviously many of these concepts are divergent from time-
honored, generally accepted ones. For instance, it is generally
considered that hemopoiesis is confined to the marrow of adult
mammals, and that lymphopoiesis describes the production of
lymphocytes. Few would agree that a primary function of lymphoid organs is to produce lymph. Lymph is looked upon, for the
most part, as a capillary filtrate (see Chap. 28). Few recognize that
a primary function of the mesenchyme and its derivatives is to
produce plasma, as well as formed elements in the blood (even
though they do so long before the liver is embryologically demarcated as a definitive organ). Presently it is held that the liver,
especially its parenchymal portion, is the principal source of the
free extracellular proteins in the plasma. Many are confounded
and remain at a loss when asked to explain the precise origin of
the plasma as a whole, or the origin of the plasma water (see Sect.
3). Only the immunoglobulins in plasma are believed to originate from lymphoid cells, and few recognize they are secreted by
clasmatosis. Current texts imply, or state categorically that plasmacytes constitute the sole source of immunoglobulins, and that the
remaining plasma proteins are of hepatic origin. With a surging
interest in immunology, most believe the function of lymphoid

organs to be principally immunologic. All have yet to fathom the true and deeper meanings of trophism!

In defense of the concepts set forth herein, it can be stated that they are definitive, yet simple. They are based on observations which can be confirmed by anyone familiar with dissection and the use of a good microscope. Singly and together they can explain many phenomena heretofore unexplainable. They can be applied to living individuals, healthy or sick, even though complicated experimental designs and tissue culture systems may supply data seemingly contradictory.

Chapter 28
LYMPHOMANIA AND CLOSING REMARKS

IN 1958, CONCLUDING his succinct review on lymphocytes, Dr. O.A. Trowell remarked, "The small lymphocyte seems a poor sort of cell, characterized by mostly negative attributes: small in size, with especially little cytoplasm, unable to multiply, dying on the least provocation, surviving *in vitro* for only a few days, living *in vivo* for perhaps a few weeks." Yet in the preface to his comprehensive treatise on the lymphocyte, published in 1967, Dr. Elves observed that, "The fascination that these cells arouse is almost unique in medical research and as evidence to this point one needs only scan the literature to see the names of a number of authors, each of whose work spans several decades: the lymphocyte creates a state of lymphomania in its adherents such as few other cells can." Alluding to a term which had been affectionately applied to himself, Dr. H. S. Mayerson mentioned in his opening address at the Second International Congress of Lymphology, held in March, 1968, that: "Lymphomania is obviously infectious and contagious and knows no international boundaries." Such statements clearly depict the theme and discourse of the many symposia, seminars, journal articles, and books on lymphocytes, lymphoid organs, and the thymus which have appeared in the last five years. While it would seem that the recent upsurge in research on the relation of lymphocytes to tissue transplantation, malignancy, and "auto-immune disease" might have led to the coining of the term "lymphomania," review of the literature will reveal that such a state had erupted in cyclic fashion even before 1891, when Paul Ehrlich applied newly discovered aniline dyes to the characterization of lymphocytes and went on to argue with Ranvier about their ultimate fate (during the aftermath of the Franco-Prussian War). Such a review will reveal that, from time to time, the heat of argument concerning the lymphocyte, its function, and its geneological relationship with other blood cells has waxed so emotional that the protagonists and antagonists could be called *cyclothymic lymphomaniacs,* a compounding of terms perhaps doubly appropriate in the light of the second section of the preceding text. The term "cyclothymic" translates literally from old Greek as a "circular or cyclic spirit." The word "lymphomaniac" translates literally from Latin as a person mad with madness (see footnote p. 6). However, looking toward its Greek root word, *nymph,* not as it was used to describe mythical maidens or brides but as it became Latinized into terms such as *limpa* and *limpidus,* referring to limpid (white) water or streams, one might define cyclothymic lymphomaniacs literally as spirits cyclically mad about limpid water or streams.

In recent times, the first person to be recognized and openly called a lymphomaniac (at first irately and later endearingly) was Dr. Yoffey, who retired in 1966 from the Chair of Anatomy at the University of Bristol, England. Since his "retirement," in pursuit of the limpid streams and the elusive lymphocytes, he has migrated through California, Australia, Israel, and many places in between to publish his third exhaustive review of the literature pertinent to the subject. (See Yoffey, J.M. and Courtice, F.C.: *Lymphatics, Lymph, and the Lymphomyeloid Complex.* New York Academic Press, 1970). Acquired too late to be used as a source reference for this treatise, those critically interested should compare our books to see how many differing conclusions lymphomaniacs can draw from similar data. Comparison may render some lymphomanic or, at least, more familiar with the cyclothymes and lymphomaniacs abroad and at home.

Illustrative of lymphomania over a relatively long period of time is the full text of Dr. Mayerson's recent address (courtesy of *Lymphology,* 2:143, 1969), as follows:

---

* With publication of monumental works in 1941, 1956, and 1970, it would appear that Dr. Yoffey gives vent to his mania in 15 year cycles.

Three Centuries of Lymphatic History—an Outline*
H. S. MAYERSON

Some ten years ago, during the Christmas holidays, Mrs. Mayerson and I were invited to a cocktail party. The party was in full swing when we arrived. As we entered the room, one of my intimate friends looked up and exclaimed to the assembled guests: "Look who's here— the lymphomaniac." The label has stuck and it is in this vein that I now say to you as a lymphomaniac to fellow lymphomaniacs, many thanks for giving me the chance to "ventilate." I am properly sensible of the privilege of being with you and reviewing some of the developments regarding the lymphatic system as they have occurred over the last three centuries. Lymphomania is obviously infectious and contagious and knows no national boundaries, for otherwise it would be difficult to explain the magnificent attendance at this congress.

Where should we start our historical survey? Who first saw a lymphatic and recognized its function? This is always a difficult question to answer. There are many references in ancient Hebrew and Greek literature of swelling of the foot and other parts of the body, of elephantiasis and lymphedema, Erasistraties of Chios in Mesopotamia described "arteries containing milk," a fairly accurate description of the mesenteric lymphatics or lacteals in the third century B.C. Herophilos of Chalcedon, also writing during the same period, made interesting and reasonably accurate descriptions of lymphatics. These were forgotten and it actually took 18 centuries for the study of anatomy and physiology to become sophisticated enough to enable observers to describe and relate their findings and attempt to explain them.

The first "modern" account of lymphatic is that of Gaspar Aselli, better known by his latinized name, Asellius. He was born in Cremona, Italy in 1581, studied in Padua and later became professor of anatomy and surgery in Milan, where he also served as Surgeon-in-Chief of the Royal Army. In 1622, he discovered the lacteals. The account of the discovery as translated by Sir Michael Foster[1] deserves to be recited.

"On the 23rd of July of that year (1622) I had taken a dog in good condition and well fed, for a vivisection at the request of some of my friends who very much wished to see the recurrent nerves. When I finished this demonstration of the nerves, it seemed good to watch the movements of the diaphragm in the same dog at the same operation. While I was attempting this, and for that purpose had opened the abdomen and was pulling down with my hand the intestines and stomach gathered together in a mass, I suddenly beheld a great number of cords as it were, exceedingly thin and beautifully white,

---

* Guest lecture at the 2nd Congress of Lymphology, Miami 1968.

scattered over the whole of the mesentery and the intestine, and starting from almost innumerable beginnings. At first I did not delay, thinking them to be nerves. But presently I saw I was mistaken in this, since I noticed that the nerves belonging to the intestine were distinct from these cords, and wholly unlike them, and besides, were distributed quite separately from them. Wherefore struck by the novelty of the thing, I stood for some time silent while there came to my mind the various disputes, rich in personal quarrels no less than in words, taking place among anatomists concerning the mesaraic veins and their function. And by chance it happened that a few days before I had looked into a little book by Johannes Costaeus written about this very matter. When I gathered my wits together for the sake of the experiment, having laid hold of a very sharp scalpel, I pricked one of the cords and indeed one of the largest of them. I had hardly touched it, when I saw a white liquid like milk or cream forthwith gush out. Seeing this, I could hardly restrain my delight, and turning to those who were standing by, to Alexander Tadinus, and more particularly to Senator Septoluis, who was both a member of the great College of the order of Physicians and while I am writing this, the Medical officer of Health, 'Eureka' I exclaimed with Archimedes and at the same time invited them to the interesting spectacle of such an unusual phenomenon. And they indeed were very much struck with the novelty of the thing."

That Asellius should have exclaimed 'Eureka' seems to me to be most inappropriate, for he really wasn't looking for lymphatic vessels. Rather this was a fine example of what we now term "serendipity." Be that as it may, Asellius operated on another dog on the next day and, to his disapointment, no vessels were visible. He correctly concluded that the absence was related to time of feeding and again tried the experiment, this time on a dog recently fed, with his same friends watching, and now white vessels were again visible.

Asellius' discovery was unquestionably exciting. It was also disconcerting, for the facts needed to be explained and fitted into current Galenic concepts. Asellius concluded that chyle was absorbed by the vessels and then transported to the liver. Chyle was "white" blood which the liver transformed into red blood.

Asellius' findings were published posthumously through the generosity of Nicholas Peiresc in 1627.[2] As Fulton[3] points out, the plates accompanying this tract are the first colored anatomical illustrations of importance in the history of bookmaking. It may be of interest that the same Nicholas Peiresc, who was the Principal Court Judge of Aix-en-Provence, confirmed Asellius' findings in man. He had a condemned criminal fed before execution and on autopsy some 90 minutes later found lacteals filled with chyle.

Recall that William Harvey had announced his discovery of the circulation on April 17, 1616—a week before Shakespeare's death—at his Lumlean Lecture to the College of Physicians in London, but his experiments were not published until 1628. Asellius could not have been aware of Harvey's concepts, but Harvey, on the other hand, probably knew of Asellius' work published the previous year and certainly knew of it later. But Harvey, in spite of his brilliance and deep insight, could not divorce himself completely from Galen and, to his dying days, maintained that lymphatics were merely veins which carried white blood to the liver.

Asellius' discovery, of itself, was perhaps not of prime importance, for it remained an isolated bit of knowledge until 1651, when Jean Pecquet, a French physician who practiced first in Dieppe and later in Paris, published his *Experimenta nova anatomica* and made known experiments he had performed as a medical student in Montpellier.[4] He had opened the thoracic cavity of a dog and removed the heart and noticed a large quantity of thin whitish fluid escape from the stump of the superior vena cava. At first, he supposed that an abcess had been opened; but he noted that upon compressing the abdomen, the flow of fluid increased. Further experiments enabled Pecquet to accurately describe the cisterna chyli and its continuation as the thoracic duct. He showed that Asellius' lacteals pour their contents into the receptacle and that the thoracic duct pours its contents into the venous system at the junction of the jugular and subclavian veins. In the following year, 1651, Johannes van Horne, Professor of Anatomy in Leyden, independently made the same discovery in man as he was performing an autopsy.

As Foster[1] has pointed out, "By this discovery of the thoracic duct and its entrance into the veins, a wholly new aspect was given to Asellius' original observation. The mere existence of special vessels such as the lacteals in the mesentery was quite consistent with, indeed supported the old view of the circulation. Pecquet's observations were wholly inconsistent with them; but between Asellius and Pecquet, Harvey's book had appeared; and it may be taken as a proof of how profoundly Harvey's arguments had in so short a time influenced men's minds, that Pecquet's observations, which if put forward thirty years before would have been rejected as impossible, were now accepted without misgivings. Indeed they afforded no little support to the new theory of circulation."

Further support was supplied at the same time by Olaus Rudbeck. This was a remarkable man. He went to the University of Upsala in 1648 where he studied medicine and botany. As a medical student he worked on the lymphatic system, the details of which I shall discuss shortly. After finishing his medical course, he went to Leyden and later returned to Upsala to teach not only medicine but chemistry, astronomy, mathematics, architecture and music. In 1661 at the age of 31 he was made Rector of the University but found time to contribute extensively to the field of botany as well as to write a historical monograph in which he attempted to prove the antiquity of Swedish culture.[5]

Rudbeck's interest in the lymphatic system was stimulated in 1650 by his observation of a whey-like fluid present near the supraclavicular notch in a calf that was being butchered. He then began a series of experiments which eventually involved the use of almost 400 animals (cats, dogs, calves, sheep, goats and wolves). In these experiments, he discovered the lymphatic plexus of the colon and rectum and he traced these structures to the cisterna chyli and showed that the vessels described by Asellius, originating in the spleen, liver and bowel wall, also empty their contents into the cysterna chyli. Influenced by Harvey, he traced the course and flow in lymphatics all over the body ligating the lymphatic vessels and watching them distend below and collapse above the ligatures. His chief contribution, like that of Harvey's, is that he really showed the lymphatic system as being a second "circulation," that flow of lymph was away from tissues and that lymph eventually returned to the bloodstream via the thoracic duct. Incidentally, he emphasized that the liver was in no way involved in the formation of blood. It was Rudbeck, too, who gave one of the most succinct descriptions of the difficulties in working with the lymphatics, difficulties only too well known to many of us. He wrote, in 1653, as follows:

"Of the many structures difficult to find in anatomical dissections, these vessels, I must confess, are by no means the least. For usually they will not tolerate the finest blunt probe, a sharp knife, a suction tube, or any other instrument whatever. And even though abundantly present, they are often obscured by fat or are overlooked if not at the moment filled with fluid, when seen they may disappear if not ligated. Thus in elusiveness they rival the lacteals and must be handled with utmost care."

I shall not go into detail about the controversy that developed at this time as to whether Rudbeck should receive the credit for having "discovered" the lymphatic system or whether Thomas Bartholinus deserves priority. Bartholinus was professor of anatomy in Copenhagen. Influenced by the work of Pecquet, he made numerous observations on the anatomy of the thoracic duct and lacteals. He eventually came to the same conclusions as did Rudbeck, denying the function of the liver in blood formation. The controversy was an example of lymphomania at its worst, with accusations of plagiarism and considerable other invective. In retrospect, both investigators contributed considerably to our knowledge of the lymphatic system and should share the honors and our respect.

We now move about a century for distinct progress in the field—to the work of William Hunter and his pupils. During this century, the injection corrosion technique was developed by de Groat, Swammerdam and Ruysch and applied to the study of the lymphatic system as a supplement to the dissection technique. Antin Nuch, surgeon in the Hague, used mercury in this way, a method widely adopted by other investigators. In 1745, Lieberkühn brought the use of the microscope to the study of the origin of lymphatics in intestinal villi. As Gans points out,[6] Lieberkühn's description of their origin in the bowel wall can be found unaltered in some of our contemporary anatomy textbooks.

I agree with John Fulton[3] that the foundation of modern knowledge concerning the function of the lymphatics was laid by the Hunters, John and William, their collaborator, William Hewson and William Hunter's pupil, William C. Crinkshank. In 1784, William Hunter[7] wrote "I think I have proved that the lymphatic vessels are the absorbing vessels all over the body; that they are the same as the lacteals; and that these altogether, with the thoracic duct, constitute one great and general system, dispersed through the whole body for absorption; and this system only does absorb and not the veins; that it serves to take up, and convey, whatever is to make, or to be mixed with the blood, from the skin, from the internal cavities or surfaces whatever. This discovery gains credit daily, both at home and abroad, to such a degree that I believe we may now say that it is almost universally adopted; and if we mistake not, in a proper time, it will be allowed to be the greatest discovery, both in physiology and pathology, that Anatomy has suggested, since the discovery of the circulation." This is certainly reasonably close to our present concept of the function of the lymphatics.

In spite of Hunter's claim, however, his concepts were far from "almost universally adopted." Indeed, Magendie in his textbook on human physiology written in the early part of the nineteenth century[8] spends considerable space in describing experiments by him and others in which results were diametrically different from those of Hunter. To quote "Thus the principal experiment of a distinguished author, who is said to have seen other fluids than chyle absorbed by the lymphatic vessels appears to be, if not an illusion, at least so imperfect that no important inference can be drawn from it. The other experiments of John Hunter being less conclusive than this, I have passed them over in silence. They have been unsuccessfully repeated by Flandrin, nor have I myself been more fortunate in attempting them."

The arguments and discussion continued until after the middle of the century when Carl Ludwig, the great teacher and physiologist, and his pupils showed that it was possible to cannulate subcutaneous lymphatics and thus collect lymph from sources other than the thoracic duct. Furthermore, the course of the lymphatics could be traced by use of Berlin blue, a substance much less toxic than the tracers previously used. It was now possible to relate events in blood capillaries to lymph formation and lymph composition and Ludwig brought forth evidence which he interpreted as showing that it was formed by a process of filtration. Lymph flow was determined by differences of pressure and composition between the blood in the capillaries and the tissue fluid which accounted for exudation from the capillaries. Secondly, chemical differences between blood and tissue fluid set up osmotic interchanges through the capillary wall.[9]

But here again, there were difficulties. Increased capillary pressure as a result of venous obstruction increased lymph flow, but there was only an insignificant change when hyperemia was produced or when there were significant increases in systemic blood pressure. And thus there began another controversy between investigators who followed Ludwig's mechanistic approach and investigators who followed Heidenhain in the belief that "vital" forces were additionally involved, i.e. that there were specific substances, lymphologues, which acted specifically to increase transudation from capillaries just as diuretics increase secretion of urine by the kidney. Heidenhain maintained that the water in lymph came from the cells and fibers of the tissues rather than from the blood stream.[10] Even my old chief and mentor, Lafayette B. Mendel, got into the controversy during his sojourn in Heidenhain's laboratory in Breslau.[11] He supported Heidenhain because he found a higher concentration of NaI in thoracic duct lymph than in the blood. Heidenhain and his pupils had also found a higher concentration of sugar and NaCl in lymph than in the blood.

The controversy was finally put to rest by the brilliant, painstaking work of Starling during the latter part of the last and early part of this century. Step by step he examined the work of the "vitalistic" school and by careful experiments pointed out the flaws in reasoning of Heidenhain and his group. His results are summarized in his Herter lectures given in New York in 1908 and published in the historic monograph entitled *The Fluids of the Body*.[11] I should remind you that Starling went to work with Heidenhain in Breslau in 1892 and while there, went along with Heidenhain's explanations and concepts. It was only after his return to England and much repetition and refinement of the Breslau experiments that he came to doubt the interpretation of his results. In 1896, he discovered the missing factor in support of Ludwig's filtration hypothesis—the colloid osmotic pressure of the plasma proteins. It had been previously supposed that the osmotic pressure of proteins, being so insignificant compared to that of salts, must be of no account in physiological processes. Starling showed the reverse to be true since the capillary is impermeable to proteins. He set to work to measure the osmotic pressures of the proteins in serum and found them to be, though small, of the order of magnitude of the capillary pressure. The problem was solved. The hydrostatic pressure and the osmotic pressure supplied the balance of forces necessary to explain the experimental observations.

Time does not permit a detailed account of how Starling, blow by blow, demolished his opponent's arguments. But it is difficult to resist some of his quips such as "I would point out at the onset that we are not justified in assuming an unknown cause so long as phenomena can be explained by a cause which is familiar to us." And further "To call in vital activity as a sort of irresponsible deity to explain irregularities in our experimental results is an unscientific and I might say cowardly device."

Starling began his fourth Herter Lecture as follows: "Under the term internal media of the body we include three distinct fluids, all of which may be regarded as derived from the original coelonic fluid. These are:

1. The circulating blood, contained in a closed system of tubes and everywhere separated from the tissues by a layer of endothelium.

2. The lymph, also contained in a closed system of endothelial tubes connected at one or more points with the blood vascular system.

3. The tissue fluid, filling all the spaces of the body and in immediate contact with the tissue cells.

This last named is the real internal medium of the body, into which the cells discharge their waste products and from which they derive their sustenance as well as their necessary oxygen."

In boldly asserting that the lymphatic system was a closed system of tubes, he denied the concept of von Reklinghausen that the lymphatics opened into the tissue spaces and firmly aligned himself with another stalwart, Florence Sabin who, in 1911[13] wrote "Lymphatics are modified veins. They are vessels lined by an endothelium which is derived from the veins. They invade the body as do blood vessels and grow into certain constant areas; their invasion of the body is, however, not complete, for there are certain structures which never receive them. The lymphatic capillaries have the same relation to tissue spaces as have blood capillaries. None of the cavities of the mesoderm, such as the peritoneal cavity, the various bursae and serous capillaries, forms any part of the lymphatic system. The lymphatic endothelium, once formed, is specific. Like blood vessels the lymphatics are for the most part closed vessels."

Rusznyak, Földi and Szabo in their monograph on Lymphatics and

Lymph Circulation[14] have reviewed the controversies regarding the origin of lymphatics and their embryological development. They aptly conclude:

"It was the appearance of Sabin's work that released the long debate of American anatomists about the evolution of lymphatics, a debate which gave rise to nearly a hundred publications without leading the problem essentially nearer to a solution and without succeeding in inducing any of the opposing parties to revise their attitude." This is but another example of the peculiarities of lymphomaniacs.

We have now arrived at the time of the first World War and its aftermath when science marched forth as never before. Work on the lymphatic system was no exception. The introduction of polyethylene tubing facilitated cannulation of lymphatics. New dyes and advances in radiological techniques made visualization more feasible in experimental animals and patients. The introduction of isotopes made possible more definitive studies on exchange between capillaries and lymphatics. The electron microscope gave us a better idea of intimate structure. It would be presumptuous of me to attempt to even summarize the progress in the last several decades. Many of you have contributed to this progress. But I would be remiss if I did not conclude with some mention of Cecil K. Drinker, for it was he who aroused my interest (and I suspect that of many others) in the lymphatic system. As a young instructor, I had the assignment of developing a laboratory course in physiology for medical students. Having read Drinker's publications later summarized by him and Fields in the monograph on Lymphatics, Lymph and Tissue Fluid published in 1933,[15] I decided it would be good to devise a laboratory experiment on lymph. The first step was to learn to cannulate the thoracic duct in the dog. This was a frustrating experience but I finally arrived at the point when I could cannulate it 4 out of 5 times and so for some 30 years, I, like Asellius and Rudbeck, demonstrated with enthusiasm the effect of various experimental procedures on lymph flow to my friends, students—in fact to anyone who would stop and listen. In retrospect, however, I perhaps missed something in not having as illustrious auditors as did Asellius and Rudbeck—I did not ask my Congressmen and Senators to watch me demonstrate.

Drinker, as you recall, maintained that the principal function of the lymphatic system was to return to the blood stream protein which had leaked from blood capillaries. His evidence was presumptive and derived chiefly from differences in protein concentration in lymph and serum. In the early forties, with the advent of isotopes, I was able to label the serum proteins with radioactive iodine and show directly that lymph protein originated chiefly from the blood stream.[16] It was my privilege and good fortune to discuss this data with Dr. Drinker

shortly before his death and to witness his pleasure in this con-
firmation of his concepts.

I have given you episodes in the history of the lymphatic system
this afternoon from the point-of-view of a physiologist. There is much
more of interest to tell about the subject. Hopefully, programs of
future Congresses will reserve time for the immunologist, the clinician
and other specialists to continue the recitation of the exciting development of concepts regarding the function of the lymphatic system in
health and disease.

Again, my thanks to you for the honor and privilege of being here.
Lymphology has come of age. Much important history is being made
by all of you. Good luck and may your lymphomania persist and
intensify to the benefit of all mankind.

References

1. Foster, M.: Lectures on the history of physiology. University Press,
   1901.

2. Aselli, G.: *De lactibus sine lacteis venis, quarto vasorum mesarai-
   corum genere, novo invento.* Dissertatis qua sententiae
   anatomicae multae uel parum perceptae illustratur. Mediolani,
   J. B. Bidellum, 1627.

3. Fulton, J. F.: *Selected Readings in the History of Physiology.*
   Thomas, Springfield, 1930.

4. Pecquet, J.: *Experimenta nova anatomica quibus incoguitum
   hactemus chyli receptaculum, et ab co per thoracem in ramos
   usque sub clabious vasa lactae detegunter.* Seb. Cramoisy and
   Gab. Cramoisy, Paris 1951.

5. Nielsen, A. E.: A translation of Olaf Rudbeck's nova exercitatis
   anatomica. *Bull. Hist. Med., 11* (1942), 304.

6. Gans, H.: On the discovery of the lymphatic circulation. *Angiology,
   13* (1962), 530.

7. Hunter, W.: Two introductory lectures to his last course of
   anatomical lectures at his theatre in Windmill St. Johnson,
   London, 1784.

8. Revere, J.: *An Elementary Treatise on Human Physiologie par
   F. Magendie,* 5th ed., 1838, Harper and Brothers, 1844.

9. Ludwig, C.: *Lehrbuch der Physiologie des Menschen.* Winter,
   Leipzig, 1858.

10. Heidenhain, R.: Versuche und Fragen zur Lehre von der Lymph-
    bildung. *Pflügers Arch. Ges. Physiol., 49* (1891), 209.

11. Mendel, L. B.: On the passage of sodium iodide from the blood to
    the lymph, with some remarks on the theory of lymph forma-
    tion. J. Physiol. 19 (1895), 227.

12. Starling, Ernest H.: *The Fluids of the Body.* Keener and Com-
    pany, Chicago.

13. Sabin, F. R.: A critical study of the evidence presented in several recent articles on the development of the lymphatic system. *Anat. Rec., 5* (1911), 417.

14. Rusznyak, I., M. Földi, and G. Szabo: *Lymphatics and Lymph Circulation.* Pergamon Press, New York, 1960.

15. Drinker, C. K. and E. Field: *Lymphatics, lymph and tissue fluid.* Williams and Wilkins Company, Baltimore, 1933.

16. Wasserman, K., H. S. Mayerson: Dynamics of lymph and plasma protein exchange. *Cardiologia (Basel), 21* (1952), 296.

Scrutiny of Dr. Mayerson's outline will reveal that several, including Asselius, Rudbeck, Hunter, and Hewson, had notions concerning the trophic function of lymphoid elements, such as those set forth in this text. To Heidenhain should be accorded credit for conceiving of lymph formation as a vital process, even though he did not single out the intestinal lymphoid tissue and its vital role in the production of chyle. Although Ludwig's mechanistic concept of lymph formation was confirmed by Starling, Drinker, Mayerson, and others who showed that plasma proteins filter into lymphatics, their studies shed relatively little light on where the plasma and its proteins are produced and where they are ultimately disposed. All of the latter assumed (as it is still assumed today) that the liver produces all the plasma proteins other than immunoglobulins (therefore, 90-95% of the plasma proteins), an assumption based on clinical studies in hospitalized individuals who failed to eat sufficient protein, failed to drink pure water, and imbibed too much alcohol, instead; and on the complicated isotope studies summarized critically in Chapter 25, p. 359. Relatively few seem to consider that some plasma proteins (and other plasma constituents) are normally reutilized for growth in the extravascular tissues which the vascular system has developed to serve (see Chap. 25, D, 5). If the bulk were to filter only into the lymphatics, one would have a situation wherein the plasma proteins cycle round and round endlessly for no obvious purposes other than immunologic and to maintain osmotic pressure in the vascular system.

Although Sabin identified the mesenchyme as the original source of the plasma (see Chap. 24, B), her description of the origin of lymphatic endothelium from venous endothelium undoubtedly led to the concept that the blood and lymph vascular systems are lined entirely by endothelium and led secondarily to the concept that lymph is formed primarily by filtration instead of secretion. Another venerable lymphomaniac, Kampmeier, pointing to the local mesenchymal origin of lymphatic endothelium, has argued seemingly in vain against Sabin's position on lymphatic origin for at least 40 years (see Kampmeier, O. F.: *The Evolution and Comparative Morphology of the Lympatic System.* Springfield, Thomas, 1969,). Though many realize that sinusoidal endothelium differs from common vascular endothelium, relatively few seem to take the differences into account insofar as filtration is concerned. Moreover, it remains to be recognized that gaps between endothelial cells expose mesenchymal tissues to the lumen, especially in the lacteals and peripheral radicles of the lymphatic system. Exposed thus, the mesenchymal tissues reside in an appropriate position to either filter or secrete large molecules into the lumen.

Thus we have touched upon some of the arguments and madness which have erupted cyclically over many years. Each point of argument obviously contains truth or it would not have withstood such a test of time. Compromising, one might suggest respectfully, that a fundamental function of the lymphatic apparatus is to filter as well as produce lymph, a limpid fluid which consists of relatively large quantities of plasma and a relatively small quantity of cells (as compared with the blood). The apparatus also conveys this fluid to the bloodstream to constitute white liquid in the blood. Without this white liquid portion, called blood plasma, the red portion of the blood containing heme would be unable to flow and therefore be relatively useless in the transport of oxygen and other essential substances. Since the blood consists of white and red portions, we may stand like Prof. Rudbeck on the point of emphasizing "that the liver is in no way involved in the formation of blood," albeit greatly concerned with its destruction, and reconstitution of many of the small molecules from which the plasma and blood cells are produced in many areas of the body.

We next look upon the ground substance and nodular masses

of cells which constitute lymphoid tissues. Although Drinker did not consider the lymphoid tissues to be quantitatively important sources of plasma or that portion of lymph which is devoid of cells, he deserves great credit for defining the lymphatic apparatus as a whole and for emphasizing the constant interposition of nodes in the lymph stream such that they are fed by the peripheral lymphatics on the one hand and, on the other, feed central lymphatics which pour into the bloodstream. Many ancient cytologists whose names are almost impossible to trace but who compounded terms such as "lymphoblasts" (precursors of lymph), "plasmablasts" (precursors of plasma), "clasmatocytes" (fragmenting cells), and "trephocytes" (feeding cells) to describe the lymphoid cells in terms of function remain to be credited for pointing to the active secretion of lymph by lymphoid cells.

Although seemingly devious, a study of the derivation and literal meaning of certain medical terms may lead to a better understanding of what these terms really mean in relation to the scheme of the body. The lymphocyte (lymph cell), perhaps, stands out as a notable exception. Is this cell "mad," or is it "limpid"? Like the cyclothyme, does it vacillate or cycle between such extremes? Perhaps, only such a "poor sort of cell, characterized by mostly negative attributes," during its life span is capable of performing many functions, singly and in combination, such as:

1. To produce quantities of plasma which mechanically carry their smaller forms, as well as other formed elements through the lymph and blood circulation.

2. To produce plasma which transports water, salts, and various free extracellular proteins (especially globulins) to be reutilized for growth in other lymphoid and nonlymphoid tissue cells.

3. To continue production of antibodies (as well as plasma with nutritive proteins) subsequent to the plasmacytic response to previously unencountered antigenic exogenous proteins, so that the latter *henceforth* may be recognized, opsonized, and reutilized conveniently for food in host cells (along with endogenous plasma proteins).

Chapter 29

ERRATA, ADDENDA, AND AFTERTHOUGHTS

TO SHARPEN THE focus in this spring of 1972, a few comments on new data and current concepts seem appropriate.

A. B-CELLS, T-CELLS, AND FOWL-PLAY

Demonstrated very recently by immunofluorescent techniques is that 10 to 30 percent of mammalian peripheral blood lymphocytes give rise to surface immunoglobulins. The percentage increases during inflammation (especially viral) and in chronic lymphocytic leukemia. It decreases often in immunologic deficiency diseases wherein the thymus fails to develop normally. In general, the larger the peripheral blood lymphocytes, the more likely it is to find evidence of immunoglobulins at their surfaces.

Currently advocated is that such cells with surface immunoglobulins, called B-cells or B-lymphocytes, are derived from the bone marrow; that they are functionally equivalent to lymphocytes derived from the bursa of Fabricius of the neonatal chick; and that these cells are concerned primarily with humoral immunity (perhaps, as precursors of plasmacytes). The remaining 70 to 90 percent of peripheral blood lymphocytes lacking such surface immunoglobulins, called T-cells or T-lymphocytes, are believed to be thymus-derived; believed to be carriers of transplantation-related "T or theta" antigens found in mice; and are believed to be concerned primarily with cellular immunity. The B-cells and T-cells are believed to interact or cooperate in a manner which remains to be defined such that appropriate antibodies are produced toward an infinite number of exogenous and endogenous antigens. Many current hypotheses embrace the clonal selection theory from random mutations as being one of the mechanisms involved.

These currently popular concepts are based on various kinds of experimental data summarized earlier in the text, for example:

1. Comparison of the effects of extirpation of the bursa of Fabricius in the neonatal chick with those of neonatal thymectomy in chickens and in mammals (see pp. 122–125).

2. Relative rates of tritiated thymidine incorporation in bone marrow lymphocytes, as compared with those in other lymphoid organs (see pp. 126–207, esp. p. 134).

3. Phytohemagglutinin (PHA) induction of peripheral blood lymphocyte transformation into antibody producing cells (see pp. 117–122), in which studies it appears, incidentally, that the smaller lymphocytes seem to account for most of the cells which transform or, at least, lend to the specificity of the antibodies produced by transforming cells.

4. Experiments on the immunologic reconstitution of sublethally irradiated or neonatally thymectomized mice, wherein it was found that tissue suspensions from the thymus and bone marrow, together, provide the most effective method (see pp. 116, 124–125).

Current interpretations of these data as they apply to humans are open to criticism for the following reasons.

1. The bursa of Fabricius, a little nubbin of lymphoepithelial tissue found in the fowl's cloaca, is lacking in mammals and has no true evolutionary counterpart except, possibly, in the thymus, thyroid and parathyroid glands. As already mentioned (pp. 105–108), like the third branchial pouch of mammalian embryos, the cloacal bursa serves as a gill in lower vertebrate orders which live in water. Well known, of course, is that fish breathe via the gills. Less well known, perhaps, is that turtles breathe via a cloacal pouch, known as the bursa of Fabricius, when submerged (especially when hibernating). With evolution, as the aquatic vertebrate emerges from the water to walk on land, to fly, and to breathe air, the gill pouch entoderm normally invaginates, becomes stranded in the mesenchyme, and continues as the epithelial component of the thymus, thyroid, and parathyroid glands in the lower neck of birds and mammals. In fowl, a variety of birds many of which resemble turtles in that they have relatively long necks and are at home in the water as well as on

land, the gill entoderm of the bursa of Fabricius also invaginates and becomes stranded in mesenchyme to constitute the epithelial reticulum of a lymphoepithelial organ which closely resembles the mammalian and avian thymus. The extirpation of this cloacal lymphoepithelial organ in neonatal chicks was found to result in an immunologic deficiency syndrome somewhat similar to neonatal thymectomy, but it was found that antibody formation seemed affected to a greater extent than immunologic reactions involving small lymphocytes as effector cells. These findings led to the presently popular concept of a dual immunologic system consisting of a bursa-dependent portion concerned primarily with humoral immunity and a thymus-dependent portion concerned with small lymphocyte-mediated, cellular immunity. Now this concept is being extolled far and wide, even though neither a bursa of Fabricius nor a true biologic counterpart has been identified in the rectum, urinary bladder, cecum, appendix, small bowel, or bone marrow of mammals.

Although the endocrine functions of the gill entoderm derivatives can be stated clearly, that is, to produce thymosin, thyroxin, and parathormone, any serious challenge to the basis of the dual immunologic system concept must provide a reasonable explanation for the differing effects of cloacal bursectomy and thymectomy in neonatal fowl. To whit, if one considers the bursa of Fabricius as an auxiliary gill, one must expect the bursal entoderm to evolve functions similar to the entoderm of the thymus, thyroid, and parathyroid glands. While it seems obvious that the cloacal bursa entoderm evolves morphologically to resemble most closely the entoderm of the thymus, one should not be misled by the resemblance to the point of excluding thyroid-like or parathyroid-like function. Therefore, if one looks toward the "third and fourth pouch syndromes" affecting human neonates, one should expect to find something akin to cloacal bursectomy in newly hatched fowl. Analogous situations then seem apparent in lymphopenic, hypogammaglobulinemic syndromes, such as Swiss type hypogammaglobulinemia and in Bruton's syndrome. In the latter a defect in parathyroid, as well as thymic function is well documented. Perhaps, further analysis of the "third and fourth pouch syndromes" with simultaneous assay for thymus, thyroid, and parathyroid activity will prove revealing, not only in neonates but also in older individuals.

While cries of "fowl-play" or "foul end-play" may resound from the bursomaniacs now proclaiming widely the existence of B-cells and a bursa-dependent immunologic system in mammals, it was their ingenious studies on fowl cloacal pouches which prompted my belief that entodermal cells from the "vestigial" gill system remain closely linked to respiration throughout phylogeny. Taking Metcalf's and Goldstein's observations at face value, it was only a short step to suggest that thymic entodermal cells produce a hormone (thymosin) which catalyzes oxidative chain phosphorylations transferring repiratory energy into DNA synthesis in lymphocytes (see pp. 108–109). Another step, then, was to consider what becomes of the energy put in, because it must come out eventually (see pp. 255–261).

2. While it appears that marrow lymphocytes incorporate DNA precursors at a very rapid rate, so do lymphocytes in remaining lymphoid organs (as compared with cells in other body tissues). This indicates that throughout the lymphatic apparatus the lymphocytes grow at a rapid rate and, therefore, cannot enjoy a prolonged biologic life such as is postulated for many of the T-cells. Thus, one must look toward reutilization or excretion as the fate of many of the lymphocytes As the body is not ordinarily wasteful of that which it has produced, one must look more carefully toward reutilization. On the basis of reutilization and the body's natural routes of utilization of DNA precursors from ingested food one may explain the disparately rapid rate of lymphocyte growth in the marrow as calculated by uptake of injected labeled precursors (see pp. 139–207).

3. It is not certain that lymphocyte transformation as observed *in vitro* actually takes place in the body. The transformation

phenomenon can be explained simply in terms of derepression of interphase chromatin in small lymphocytes such that, lacking repression, these cells resume DNA synthesis, reutilization of DNA from other cells, RNA synthesis, cytoplasmic globulin production, and cytoplasmic shedding of plasma containing immunoglobulins (as well as other free extracellular proteins), as outlined on pp. 117–121.

4. Suspensions of tissue obtained from the thymus not only contain relatively large numbers of small lymphocytes (or the products of their disintegration), but also contain entodermal cells capable of producing a hormone which accelerates DNA synthesis in lymphoid cells. Under the impetus of the latter reutilization (or reutilization of DNA precursors) of the former will be accelerated, irrespective of the body or the experimental system into which both are inoculated.

5. Immunologic reactions, as outlined on pp. 233–240, involve many types of cells other than those which can be identified as B-cells, T-cells, and plasmacytes. Bone marrow suspensions, although a moderately rich source of medium-sized lymphocytes, also are an excellent source of reticular stroma, macrophages, and diverse cellular material which can be reutilized in the growth of the latter. Few underestimate the importance of macrophages, but many remain to appreciate the necessity of stroma.

With this background one may provide an alternate explanation for the presence of cells possessing surface immunoglobulins and cells lacking them in the peripheral blood of mammals. For if the observations of the older histologists are correct (as outlined on pp. 35–57) as they grow in the various lymphoid organs, the lymphocytes synthesize and shed globulins to the point that most of the cytoplasm is gone by the time that the small cytoplasm-poor lymphocyte stage is reached. However, it is conceivable that many of the larger peripheral blood lymphocytes and a few of the smaller ones have been shed from the various lymphoid organs prior to complete repression of DNA synthesis, RNA synthesis, cytoplasmic globulin production, and cytoplasmic shedding. Recent studies by J. B. Hay, M. J. Murphy, Bede Morris, and M. Bessis (*Am J Path,*

66:1–42, 1972) may support this point of view. Further support may be added by the consideration that in PHA systems many of the small lymphocytes resembling T-cells, after de-repression of interphase chromatin, resume DNA synthesis, RNA synthesis, and the production of globulins having a high degree of immunologic specificity for antigens encountered by the body in the past.

Such considerations may help students of biology and medicine to formulate clearer concepts of B-cells, T-cells, and peripheral blood lymphocytes. Perhaps modern experimental biologists, like some nations, are too preoccupied with defense to worry about how populations are fed.

B. CORTISOL, THYMOSIN, AND BIOENERGETICS

Overlooked earlier, but reported recently by J. F. Whitfield, A. D. Perris, and T. Youdale (*Exp Cell Res, 52*:349–362, 1968) is that cortisol exerts its lymphocytolytic action by splitting histones from the nuclear DNA. They found this hormonal action to be phosphate-linked and oxygen-dependent, thus similar to the action of ionizing radiation. They suggested that cortisol may act on the lymphocytes by forcing metabolic reactions in the nuclear membrane to shift from their main task of transferring energy from respiration into ATP to the formation of abnormal quantities of phosphate-rich, chromatin dissociation compounds, such as phospho-proteins. Also, they mentioned that other compounds, such as PHA, valinomycin, and parathormone, cause disaggregation of chromatin structure, and share an ability to redirect respiratory energy from ATP synthesis into increased formation of phospho-proteins. Suggested earlier (p. 108 and 288) is that the thymic hormone (thymosin) may serve to catalyze oxidative chain phoshorylations leading to the synthesis of DNA in lymphocytes —thus opposing the action of cortisol. Such considerations point up the earlier stressed importance of oxygen tension, phosphate, high-energy phosphate bonds, and bioenergetics in lymphocyte metabolism.

Within the last year, as a result of Sutherland's recognition for establishing the role of cyclic AMP as an important mediator of intracellular energy and functional direction, the role of the nucleotides and polyribonucleotides have come under very intensive scrutiny. It cannot be predicted accurately at this time where lymphocytes, lymphocytolysis, and their donation of nucleic acids will bear on the problem as a whole, but they will have to be taken into account.

C. NEWER CONCEPTS OF ANTIBODIES

Quite recently, also, there has been an explosion of research and literature concerning the molecular structure and function of antibodies and complement, particularly as assessed in test tubes and experimental systems. Long known, of course, is that antibodies not only agglutinate, precipitate and opsonize, but also lyse bacteria and sensitized red cells. Recent work suggests that some of the actions of antibodies and complement are mediated through activation of adenyl cyclase and cyclic AMP—another consideration which may punctuate the importance of relatively high concentrations of polynucleotides and nucleotides in small lymphocytes. Recently it has become apparent that small lymphocytes can not only kill grafted or neoplastic cells directly, but also are associated with the production of soluble cytotoxins and a migration inhibiting factor (MIF) affecting macrophages. Moreover, it appears that the cytotoxic actions of lymphocytes can be blocked by blocking antibodies, at least *in vitro* and in small laboratory animals. Finally, it has been found in human blood that specific antibodies toward tumor specific antigens (TSA) are demonstrable, thus far notably in hepatic, bowel, and breast malignancies. Although the demonstrability of tumor specific antibodies so far correlates poorly with the patient's clinical resistence to his tumor, the finding of such antibodies proves a boon to cancer detection.

Although portions of the foregoing text may seem quite naive to those well versed in immunology, three points should be driven home here.

1. In the body the actions of agglutinins, precipitins, opsonins, lysins, cells which phagocytize, and cells which lyse other cells is ultimately the same, i.e. to reduce foreign or noxious material into forms which host cells can either reutilize for food or get rid of conveniently.

2. The humoral factors and cells which demonstrate immunologic activity are normally produced in relatively great quan-

tity, enjoy relatively short biologic lives, and are constantly being broken down and reutilized presumably for food, whether or not an overt infection or a graft is present in the body.

3. Because immunologic techniques have supplied a means to trace the production and movements of free extracellular proteins and cells in various body compartments better than we have been able to do so before, it is conceivable these techniques may pave the way to a superior understanding of normal human physiology, particularly in the realms of nutrition and control of growth.

D. IMMUNOSUPPRESSION

Recently reported clinical successes with immunosuppressive therapy in renal transplantation and in some of the poorly understood mesenchymal diseases, such as rheumatoid arthritis, systemic lupus, and ulcerative colitis, seem to belittle the rationale and side effects of immunosuppression as outlined on pp. 264–281. In the process of being established as a conventional therapeutic module, immunosuppression's melodramatic effectiveness seems far to outweigh less dramatic, undesirable side effects. Increased proclivity toward repeated or unusual infections seems offset by the use of appropriate antibiotics by the well-trained and alert clinicians managing immunosuppressed patients. The spectre of cancer has not yet loomed sufficiently large to offset the desirable remissions from seriously debilitating diseases under treatment. In adults whose growth rate is relatively slow in comparison with neonates, retardation of whole body growth poses no major problem. Accurate evaluation of the problems in point, therefore, will await the test of time and experience. At present it appears the capacity to obliterate memory for immunologic experience is a blessing, particularly to those severely afflicted with some of the obscure mesenchymal diseases, yet thriving (somewhat like axenic animals) under careful supervision in many medical institutions.

E. LYSOGENY

Now clear to biochemists (see A. Kornberg, *Stanford M.D.,* *11(1):*2–9, 1972) is that DNA from infective organisms is incorporated rapidly into the chromosomal DNA of infected hosts. The process of inserting heterologous DNA into the chromosomes is called *lysogeny* and *recombination*. While it remains to be determined what incites the recombined DNA to be expressed in terms of normal vs. unusual protein synthesis, growth, or in cellular destruction, recognition of the processes has opened fabulous new horizons in biology, particularly in the realms of molecular biology and genetic engineering.

In this book, instead of "lysogeny" and "recombination," the terms "hybridization," "incorporation," and "reutilization" of DNA have been used to convey meanings somewhat similar, particularly as these processes may apply between circulating lymphocytes, proliferating lymphocytes, and other kinds of rapidly growing cells in the same individual; or between donor lymphocytes and rapidly growing lymphoid cells in an unrelated recipient (see pp. 116, 120, 212-217 and see "reutilization" in index). Important, of course, are the therapeutic applications of these naturally occurring phenomena. At present, Lawrence's transfer factor obtained from small lymphocyte dialyzates shows great promise in young individuals congenitally lacking in thymic development and the power to overcome various infections. In a variety of clinical situations, perhaps, infusions of lymphocyte concentrates or their disintegration products will prove beneficial between suitably matched individuals, one of whom acutely requires the substrate, information, or power contained in the lymphocytes of the other.

F. REVERSE TRANSCRIPTASES

It is now accepted, as shown by Temin, that viral RNA can function as a *reverse transcriptase,* or *template* which imprints new informational codes on the DNA of growing mammalian cells. With new codes, the infected cells may proceed to show abnormal chromosomes, grow abnormally, or become neoplastic. This spring, Heller *et al.* showed in mice (see *Blood* 39:453-471, 1972) that transplanted plasmacytomas may induce change in immunoglobulins produced in lymphocytes, such that those at the surface of circulating "B-cells" become diminishingly "polyclonal" (heterogeneous) and increasingly "monoclonal" (homogeneous) with Fab fragments characteristic of abnormal globulins in animals donating the plasmacytomas. In addition, they showed that purified RNA from the neoplastic donor plasmacytes induces such changes. These findings perhaps punctuate the importance of RNA from endogenous plasmacytes as normal sources of reverse transcriptases (see pp. 239, 389) and precipitate some important questions, such as

1. In healthy mammals, are the relatively small number of plasmacytes in hemopoietic organs really the continuing source of relatively large quantities of immunologically specific globulins?

2. Or, as a function of their relatively great cytoplasmic RNA production, are they quantitatively important sources of reverse transcriptases which continually modulate normal and immune globulin production in the enormous population of lymphocytes and other mononuclear cells normally growing and shedding cytoplasm in the reticulum of many lymphoid organs?

G. WHAT IS LYMPH?

Realizing that lymphocytes and other lymphoid cells not only release globulins but also secrete plasma by shedding cytoplasm, it seems cogent to close with an inclusive definition of lymph. Grossly, it is the variably turbid, sometimes milky fluid consisting of plasma and mononuclear cells which flows via lymphatics to replete the colorless liquid in circulating blood. It originates as the composite of plasma and mononuclear cells shed from lymphoid organs into ultrafiltrates made up of water and diverse larger molecules which emanate in variable quantities from peripheral parenchymal cells and circulating blood. It supplies the circulating blood with water, trophic proteins, and smaller nutritive molecules, and with cells which not only feed but also immunologically maintain *morphostasis* in peripheral tissues. In addition, it serves to carry relatively large molecules excreted from growing peripheral tissue cells and invading microorganisms onward to lymphoid organs where they can be reutilized for nutritive and immunologic purposes, or to nonlymphoid organs where they can be excreted conveniently.

It is hoped that this kinetic definition, along with diverse basic considerations set forth earlier, will prove valuable to those seeking clearer insights into normal and pathologic physiology, and into the relatively embryonic science of lymphology. Moreover, it is hoped these clearer insights will lead to better prevention and treatment of iatrogenic and naturally occurring diseases.

Chapter 30

GENERAL SUMMARY

F EW TOPICS IN medicine are so shrouded in mystery, but of such fundamental importance as the function of *lymphoid organs, lymphocytes, and lymph.* Altogether comprising 2 to 3 percent of total body weight in mammals, these *lymphoid elements,* respectively, constitute the most rapidly grown, turned over, and fluid of all tissues in the body. While it is established that these elements subserve important immunologic functions, it is the purpose of this book to show that *their function, basically, is to feed other cells in the body.*

In the first section of the text, anatomic and microscopic observations are outlined to indicate that *the mass of mononuclear lymphoid cells normally feeds other cells by two mechanisms:*

1. By *shedding cytoplasm* which, in turn, dissolves to yield *plasma.* In aqueous solution this plasma transports diverse large and small molecules through the vascular system to nourish various tissues.

2. By *migrating* passively within the circulating *plasma* in compact forms, such as *small lymphocytes.* Leaving the *plasma,* the latter proceed to *migrate actively* into cells of other tissues to *donate* residual protoplasm (principally *nucleoplasm*) . Via this route relatively large nondiffusible molecules, such as DNA, are transported to growing cells in other tissues at rates more rapid than these molecules can proceed via diffusion.

Particular emphasis is placed on gel-sol relationships; and how *lymphoid organs,* in producing both plasma and lymphocytes, *actually secrete lymph.* As functions of their vascular and extravascular sources of substrate, specific *trophic* (as well as immunologic) functions of various lymphoid organs and their component mononuclear cells are outlined tentatively.

As this *trophic concept* remains to be accepted generally, in the second section the thymus gland is used as a key to unlock several compartments of the lymphoid tissue—lymphocyte mystery. Anatomic data are integrated with data from tissue culture, isotope labeling and immunologic experiments to indicate that the *thymus normally feeds* remaining lymphoid tissues with relatively large quantities of *thymocyte DNA* and an *entodermal hormone* which accelerates DNA synthesis in lymphocytes. Stimulated by the thymic hormone, remaining lymphoid organs reutilize the thymocyte DNA to accelerate lymphopoiesis and perform their designated trophic functions at accelerated rates. Particularly emphasized are the thymic "priming" of other lymphoid tissues during the neonatal period, and the active role of intestinal lymphoid tissue in producing chyle during the absorption of food.

Pointing to *lymphocyte DNA as a relatively concentrated source of important molecular substrate, genetic information, and nucleoside-bound phosphate bond energy,* discussion of the second section is devoted to the profound biologic and clinical implications of *lymphocytolysis* and *DNA donation* in relation to growth, stress, repair of tissue injury, and immunologic reactions. Emphasized here and throughout is that the *immunologic function of lymphoid elements is fundamentally trophic,* the opsonic action of antibodies and the lytic action of sensitized lymphocytes being specialized, respectively, to reduce antigens and living foreign material into simple nontoxic forms which can be reutilized conveniently for food in host cells.

The third section of the text is devoted to review of the development of the hemopoietic and vascular systems as they relate to one another, and as both relate to the feeding of remaining tissues. Emphasized are:

1. How the *plasma* produced by cytoplasmic shedding from mononuclear lymphoid cells enables formed elements, free extracellular proteins, and many kinds of smaller molecules to *flow* into and through the vascular system.

2. How the *flow* of whole blood and lymph thus differentiated *induces vascular differentiation* in proportion to the flow rate locally established.

3. How *mononuclear lymphoid cells constitute the principal source of plasma and its proteins,* both *before* and *after* the

liver and its parenchymal cells are demarcated embryologically.

The fourth section of the text presents a new concept of mesenchymal development and function—the supportive, hemopoietic, vasoformative, and nutritive functions being considered simultaneously. Next, to emphasize that the lymphoid derivatives of mesenchyme are specialized to *secrete,* as well as *filter* lymph, older concepts of lymph production are reviewed critically. Finally, *lymphomania* is defined and illustrated to clear the way for filling "one of the most disgraceful and humiliating gaps in all medical knowledge."

INDEX